AF522054

About the Author : A leading authority on nutrition and holistic therapies with a Ph.D. in Food Science and Nutrition, **Dr. (Mrs.) Jyoti Singh,** is presently attached with Government Home Science College, Chandigarh. She has been writing various articles in nutrition for Hindustan Times and Times of India. Her articles have appeared in many renowned journals like Journal of Research, SKUAST-J, Himachal Journal of Agricultural Research, Beverage and Food World, and Journal of Dairying, Foods & Home Sciences to name a few. Adding to her credit is the research on soybean and Dr. Jyoti has been successful in bringing out several important features of soybean paneer (Tofu) into the limelight. Being a bright student right through her academic phase, she has won various scholarships for her B.Sc., M.Sc. and Ph.D. She also has two gold medals to her credit. Dr. Jyoti had a major breakthrough in her research when she worked on food consumption behaviour and nutrient adequacy of army personnel in selected cantonment areas.

About the Book : Diet and nutrition is an important part of health-care, at times much more than medicine and treatment, and in the present-day extremely health-conscious society, an authoritative book on the subject is most welcome. Though this work by an expert is aimed at the student of Dietetics, it is equally useful for the general reader because it is neither very elementary nor painfully technical, maintaining a balance between the two. In it the basic dietetic information is suitably documented and the scientific as well as practical aspects are commendably integrated.

Students and professionals of Home Science, Dietetics, Nutrition, Nursing and Medical or Para-medical courses, will find the book most useful; it covers all the diseases in quite some detail and food-planning needed in their treatment.

Handbook
of
Nutrition and Dietetics

Published by :
Lotus Press Publishers & Distributors

FROM THE DIETITIAN'S DESK

Handbook of Nutrition and Dietetics is an extremely well written and lucid discussion of most of the disorders requiring dietary modifications. It is a well documented source of basic diet information and presents a commendable integration of technical as well as the practical aspects. With the vision and clarity of organisation of contents, this handbook, I am sure, will prove to be a convenient reference and guide for both students and professionals alike.

Ms. Manju Mathur, RD

Chief Dietician and Head
Department of Dietetics
Government Medical College and Hospital
Sector-32, Chandigarh

President
Indian Dietetic Association
Chandigarh

Handbook of Nutrition and Dietetics

Dr. Jyoti Singh

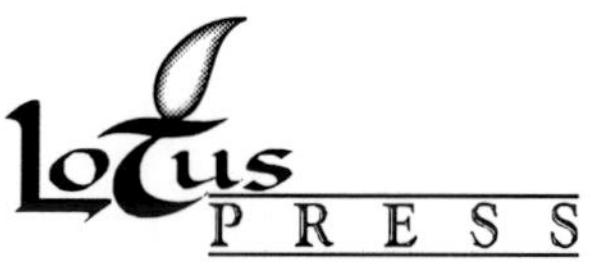

4735/22, Prakash Deep Building
Ansari Road, Darya Ganj,
New Delhi - 110002

Lotus Press : Publishers & Distributors
Unit No. 220, 2nd Floor, 4735/22, Prakash Deep Building,
Ansari Road, Darya Ganj, New Delhi- 110002
Ph.: 41325510, 98118-38000
• E-mail : lotuspress1984@gmail.com
www.lotuspress.co.in

Handbook of Nutrition and Dietetics

ISBN: 81-8382-151-0

Printed & Published by : **Lotus Press Publishers & Distributors,** New Delhi-02

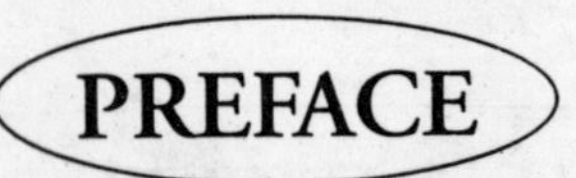

This book has been written as a text for courses on food sci nutrition, dietetics, nursing, students of home science, agricu hotel management and practicing dieticians. Health cons people can gain an insight into nutrition and dietetics, which an important role in our daily life. This book illustrates the g principles of nutrition and diet therapy, which are involved i planning.

If the students and other readers could find this book inter and helpful then I would consider my efforts to have been aw I request my teacher friends as well as the students to point c mistakes, if any and send their comments and suggestions f further improvement of this book.

E-mail ID: drjyoti.singh@gmail.com

Main Features:

- Review questions at the end of the chapter help re knowledge and understanding.
- Key terms highlighted within the text.
- Text boxes draw special attention to important issues
- Illustrated throughout.

—

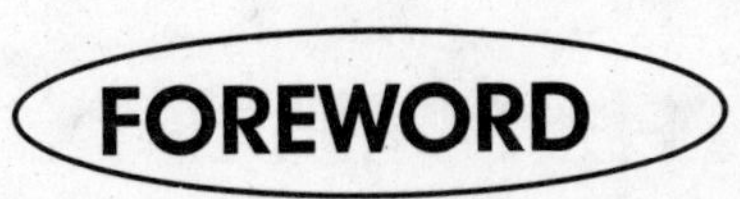

I am very happy to note that Dr. Jyoti Singh has brought out this publication entitled "*Handbook of Nutrition and Dietetics*". It fills the gap between elementary books containing little scientific explanation and advanced books which examine the subject in detail but are only suitable for those who have a comprehensive scientific training.

In this book an attempt has been made to convey basic scientific factors and principles necessary for the understanding of basic and therapeutic nutrition.

This book will be an asset for the students of Home Science, Nutrition, Dietetics, Nursing and Medical/Paramedical courses, as it presents the latest knowledge along with practical approach in dealing with different disease conditions.

I congratulate Dr. Jyoti Singh for having done a splendid service to the student community.

Ms. Damandeep
Head
Department of Foods and Nutrition
Govt. Home Science College
Chandigarh

CONTENTS

Carbohydrates

Carbohydrates are the most abundant organic compounds in nature and the chief source of energy for the human body. These are made up of carbon, hydrogen and oxygen. Carbohydrates are manufactured inside plants from carbon dioxide in the air and water, under the influence of sunlight. The basic building blocks of all carbohydrates are sugar molecules.

Photosynthesis: In the presence of sunlight, a green plant takes carbon dioxide from the air and combines it with water to form carbohydrate compounds (sugars)

a. $CO_2 + H_2O \rightarrow$ (light) $\rightarrow$ carbohydrates + O_2

b. The energy of the sunlight is locked up as chemical energy in the sugars

Classification of Carbohydrates

Carbohydrates are classified in various ways.

(1) Simple and Complex Carbohydrates

Carbohydrates can be classified into simple and complex carbohydrates according to their molecular or biological structure. Simple carbohydrates (or "simple sugars") include monosaccharides and disaccharides; and complex carbohydrates (or "complex sugars"), include oligosaccharides and polysaccharides.

Simple carbohydrates: These are easily digested by the body and are found in many fruits. They are often found in processed foods usually food products containing refined sugar.

Complex carbohydrates: These are found in nearly all plant-based foods, and usually take longer for the body to digest. They are most commonly found in bread, pasta, rice and vegetables.

(2) Sugars, Starches and Dietary Fiber

Carbohydrates are sometimes classified into sugars, starches and dietary fiber (non-starch polysaccharides). Generally, sugars are "simple carbohydrates", while starches and dietary fiber are "complex carbohydrates".

(3) High and Low Glycemic Index Carbohydrates

The classification of carbohydrates into "simple" or "complex carbohydrates" has been superseded by the glycemic index, which means that how quickly they raise the blood sugar levels. The glycemic index divides carbohydrate-containing foods into high, medium or low glycemic index foods. Most sugars or sugary carbohydrates (except fructose, or fruit sugar) are classified as high-glycemic-index foods and should (for best effects on blood-sugar and insulin sensitivity) be eaten in moderation—preferably in combination with low glycemic index foods.

(4) Refined or Unrefined Carbohydrates

Carbohydrates can also be classified into refined or unrefined carbohydrates, depending on their processing by the food manufacturers. Sugars are one of the most common ingredients in processed foods.

(5) Available and Unavailable Carbohydrates

Carbohydrates are often classified as available and unavailable carbohydrates. Available carbohydrates are those that can be hydrolyzed by enzymes of the human gastrointestinal system to monosaccharides that are absorbed in the small intestine and enter the pathways of carbohydrate metabolism. Unavailable

Composition of Carbohydrate Sugars	
Type of Carbohydrate	**Molecular Contents**
Monosaccharides	
Glucose (basic sugar unit)	1 molecule of glucose
Fructose (fruit sugar)	1 molecule of fructose
Galactose(derived from lactose)	1 molecule of galactose
Disaccharides	
Sucrose (table sugar)	1 molecule of glucose + 1 molecule of fructose
Maltose (malt sugar)	2 molecules of glucose
Lactose (milk sugar)	1 molecule of galactose + 1 molecule of glucose
Oligosaccharides	Maltodextrin
Polysaccharides	Starch: amylose, amylopectin, Non-starch: cellulose, pectins

carbohydrates are not hydrolyzed by endogenous human enzymes, although they may be fermented in the large intestine to varying extents.

Simple and Complex Carbohydrates

(1) Monosaccharides

The simplest carbohydrates are monosaccharides, which are small straight-chain aldehydes and ketones with many hydroxyl groups added, usually one on each carbon except the functional group.The word monosaccharide comes from mono, meaning "one", and saccharide, meaning "sugar". Common monosaccharides are **glucose** (also called dextrose), **fructose**, and **galactose**. Monosaccharides are a type of carbohydrate. Except for fructose, they are typically high on the glycemic index, which means that, when digested, they cause a rapid rise in blood-glucose levels.

Glucose (derived from the Greek word for "sweet") is the primary form of sugar stored in the human body for energy. Probably the most common source of glucose is table sugar (sucrose). Glucose is also obtained from starch, the major storage form of carbohydrate in plants.

Structure of Glucose

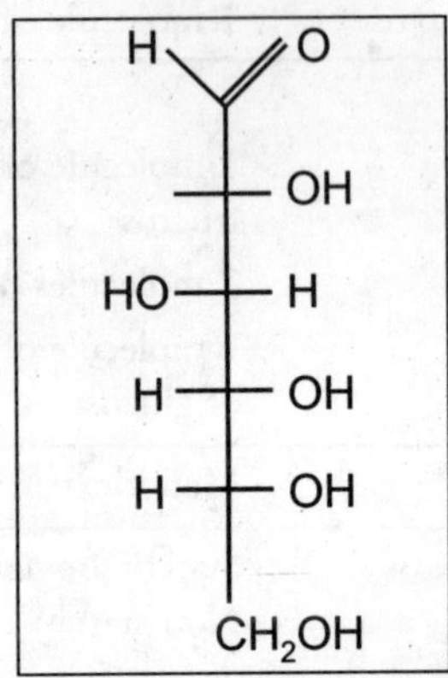

Fructose (fruit sugar) as name indicates, is found in fruits and its sources include fruits, honey and high-fructose corn syrup.

Galactose comes from lactose in milk. After being absorbed by the body, fructose and galactose are converted into glucose by the liver and then used as fuel.

(2) Disaccharides

Disaccharides are composed of two monosaccharide units bound together by a covalent glycosidic bond. The binding between the two sugars results in the loss of a hydrogen atom (H) from one molecule and a hydroxyl group (OH) from the other. The most common disaccharides are **sucrose** (cane or beet sugar—made from one glucose and one fructose), **lactose** (milk sugar—made from one glucose and one galactose) and **maltose** (made of two glucose **molecules**). The formula of these disaccharides is $C_{12}H_{22}O_{11}$. These are also **high** on the glycemic index.

Sucrose is found in table sugar and is made up of glucose and fructose. Sucrose is the most common food sweetener. It is an easily assimilated macronutrient that provides a quick source of energy to the body, provoking a rapid rise in blood glucose upon ingestion.

Lactose comes from milk and is made up of glucose and galactose. Lactose has a complex molecular structure, and just because of that some people (lactose intolerant) are unable to digest it properly.

Maltose, or malt sugar, is a disaccharide formed from two units of glucose . Maltose can be broken down into two glucose molecules by hydrolysis. In living organisms, the enzyme maltase can achieve this very rapidly. Like Galactose, maltose is not commonly found in nature.

(3) Oligosaccharides

The term oligosaccarides is derived from "oligo"—meaning, a few—and "saccharide"—meaning, sugar. An oligosaccharide is a complex carbohydrate containing three to six units of simple sugars (monosaccharides). Oligosaccharides are typically low glycemic index carbohydrates, and help to maintain stable blood glucose levels when eaten as part of a meal. Naturally occurring oligosaccharides are found in plants. Important oligosaccharides are raffinose and stachyose. These oligosaccharides are found primarily in legumes. They cannot be digested properly by small intestine and end up being metabolized and expelled from the large intestine. Fermentation of these oligosaccharides by the intestinal microorganisms is largely responsible for the flatulence associated with consumption of legumes.

(4) Polysaccharides

Polysaccharides (sometimes called glycans) are relatively complex carbohydrates. They are the polymers made up of many monosaccharides joined together by glycosidic links. They are therefore very large, often branched, molecules. They are insoluble in water, and have no sweet taste. When all the constituent monosaccharides are of the same type they are termed homopolysaccharides; when more than one type of monosaccharide is present they are termed heteropolysaccharides. Examples include storage polysaccharides such as starch and glycogen and structural polysaccharides such as cellulose and chitin. Starch is the main polysaccharide used by plants to store glucose and is the most common form of edible polysaccharides.

(a) Starch

It is made up of a mixture of amylose and amylopectin. Amylose consists of a linear chain of several hundred glucose molecules and amylopectin is a branched molecule made of several thousand glucose units. Starches are insoluble in water. They can be digested by hydrolysis catalyzed by enzymes called amylases, which can break the alpha-linkages. Humans and other animals have amylases, so they can digest starches. Potato, rice, wheat, and maize are major sources of starch in the human diet.When humans eat starch, amylase found in the saliva and intestines, breaks down the starch and allows the glucose to be absorbed into the bloodstream. Once absorbed into the bloodstream, the human body uses insulin to disperse and distribute the glucose to areas and cells where it is needed for energy or stores it as "liquid fuel" known as glycogen.

(b) Glycogen

Glycogen, found in animal muscle tissue, is similar in structure to starch, so it is sometimes called animal starch. Glycogen is not a significant source of carbohydrate in the diet. Rather, it is a carbohydrate formed within the body's tissues and is crucial to the body's metabolism and energy balance. Glycogen is found in the liver and muscles, where it is constantly recycled (i.e. broken down to form glucose for immediate energy needs and synthesized for storage in the liver and muscles). These small stores of glycogen help sustain normal blood glucose during short-term fasting periods (e.g. sleep) and provide immediate fuel for muscle action. These reserves also protect cells from depressed metabolic function and injury.

(c) Dietary Fibre

Many foods contain non-digestible carbohydrates. These non-digestible carbohydrates are designated as "dietary fibre" or unavailable carbohydrates. Dietary fibres are structural components of plants.

A common misconception about fiber is that it is not digested by enzymes in the body and therefore provides no calories or nutrients. But the category "fibre" includes chemicals that can be dissolved, and some substances that can be digested partially. One should eat quite a complex mixture of fibers. Dietary fibres occurring in foods are of two types: Soluble fibres and Insoluble fibres

(1) Soluble Fibres

They are soluble in water and become sticky in consistency. Examples include:

Pectins

Pectins find widespread use in foods such as jams and jellies because of their ability to form stable gels. Completely esterified pectins do not require the addition of acid or electrolyte to form gels. The presence of calcium salts enhances the gelling capacity and decreases the dependence on pH and sugar concentration. Pectic substances are of importance as a component of dietary fibre because of their ion-exchange properties, due to the presence of the galacturonic acid units, and gelling (viscosity enhancing) properties.

Gums and Mucilages

Hydrocolloids (gums, mucilages) are used in small amounts in food products for their thickening (viscosity increasing), gelling, stabilizing, or emulsifying ability. They are derived from seaweed extracts, seeds, and microbial sources.

(2) Insoluble Fibres

They pass through the digestive tract largely unchanged except for being broken into smaller pieces by chewing. Examples include:

Cellulose

Cellulose is the most abundant molecule in nature and the major cell wall structural component in plants. Cellulose is an unbranched linear chain of several thousand glucose units with beta glycosidic linkages. Cellulose has been used as a bulking agent in food due to its water-absorbing ability and low solubility. Cellulose is not digested to any extent by the enzymes of the human gastrointestinal system. It is insoluble in water and is found abundantly in the bran of cereal grains.

Hemicelluloses

Hemicelluloses may be present in soluble and insoluble forms and are comprised of a number of branched and linear polysaccharides. These are found in the cell walls of many plants. Hemicelluloses are of much lower molecular weight than cellulose. Component monosaccharide units may include xylose, arabinose, galactose, mannose, glucose, glucuronic acid, and galacturonic acid. Both soluble and insoluble hemicelluloses play important roles in food products, the former functioning as soluble and the latter as insoluble fibre. They are characterized by their ability to bind water and hence serve as bulking agents. Hemicelluloses are fermented to a greater extent than cellulose in the colon.

Lignin

A wood like substance found in bran, fruit skins, nuts and whole grains.

Usefulness of Fibre in Human Body

1. Dietary fibre holds water so that the stools are soft, bulky and readily eliminated. A high fibre intake prevents or relieves constipation but the amount of fibre required for this effect varies considerably from individual to individual.
2. The large bulky stools mean dilution of the colon contents. Thus, any potential carcinogen or toxin that might be present would become diluted and be less harmful.
3. Fibre increases the motility of the small intestine and colon. It has been found to decrease the transit time. When the transit time is shortened, then there is less time for exposure of mucosa (the lining of the inside of all the hollow organs in the body) to harmful toxicants and there could be less time for bacteria to produce harmful substances.

4. Fiber has been found to delay the gastric emptying. This promotes a feeling of fullness, thus helps in keeping the energy intake within the requirement and a smoother response by blood circulation to the absorbed glucose and hence decreased insulin secretion. This is the only reason that the diabetic patients who consume high fibre diet need less insulin.
5. Pectines, mucilages and gums chelate with the bile acids. This stops the reabsorption of bile acids and thus reduces cholesterol level in circulation.

> The cellulose, hemicellulose and lignin are insoluble fibers, which can absorb and hold water in the digestive system. Whereas, pectins, mucilages and gums are soluble fibers, which are partially broken down in digestion to a gel-like substance, which also retains water.

Because of these physiological effects, fiber is considered beneficial in preventing, alleviating or curing a number of diseases and conditions, including:

- Arteriosclerosis (hardening of the arteries)
- Excess food intake
- Diverticular disease
- Irritable bowel syndrome
- Crohn's disease
- Gallstone formation
- Constipation

Sources

Recent recommendations suggest that one should get fiber from a variety of foods high in different types of fibers, rather than from dietary supplements. A healthy diet should provide a mixture of both soluble and insoluble fibers. Different sources of fibre include:

- Fruits, especially apples and citrus
- Vegetables, especially leafy green varieties

- Oats
- Wheat bran
- Whole grains
- Legumes
- Most fruits and vegetables

A good source of fiber should have at least three grams of fiber. High-fiber foods provide five grams or more.

Requirements

A healthy adult should consume 30 to 40 grams of fiber a day. Children between the ages of 3 to18 need less fiber than adults, and they need different amounts at different ages. To calculate a child's daily fiber requirements, add the child's age to the number five (for five grams). For example, a four-year-old needs nine grams of fiber a day.

Functions of Carbohydrates

Carbohydrates have many major important functions in the body:

1. Providing energy and regulation of blood glucose
2. Spare the use of proteins for energy
3. Help in preventing ketosis
4. Act as flavour and sweeteners
5. Give bulk to the diet

Classification of Carbohydrates	
Monosaccharides	Glucose, Fructose
Disaccharides	Sucrose, Lactose
Oligosaccharides	Raffinose, Stachyose, Fructo-oligosaccharides
Polysaccharides	Cellulose, Hemicelluloses, Pectins, b-Glucans, Fructans, Gums, Mucilages, Algal polysaccharides
Sugar alcohols	Sorbitol, Mannitol, Xylitol, Lactitol, Maltitol

1. Providing Energy and Regulation of Blood Glucose

Carbohydrates provide energy to the body cells. When carbohydrates are consumed, the body turns them into glucose, which provides sufficient energy for everyday tasks and physical activity. If an individual consumes more of carbohydrates, then these get stored in the liver and muscle cells as glycogen for future, when the body needs an extra burst of energy. The glycogen that isn't stored in liver and muscle cells is turned into fat. While exercising, the body first uses glycogen to be used for energy and then will turn to it's fat reserve for energy.

It's important to remember that "low-carbohydrate" doesn't mean "no-carbohydrate." Be sure to eat moderate amounts of carbohydrates to keep the body fueled properly. The body needs a certain amount of carbohydrates to function properly, and an insufficient supply can cause fatigue, muscle cramps, and poor mental function. A low-carbohydrate diet might seem healthy, but if taken to the extreme, can be very dangerous to a person's overall well-being. Each gram of carbohydrate when oxidized yields approximately 4 kcal of energy.

2. Spare the Use of Proteins for Energy

Maintaining a regular intake of carbohydrates prevents protein from being used as an energy source. Gluconeogenesis slows down and amino acids become easily available for the biosyntheses of enzymes, antibodies, receptors and other important proteins. Furthermore, an adequate amount of carbohydrates will prevent the degradation of skeletal muscle and other tissues such as the heart, liver, and kidneys.

3. Help in Preventing Ketosis

For the normal oxidation of fats some carbohydrate is necessary. In the absence of adequate carbohydrate large amounts of ketone bodies are produced. The accumulation of ketone bodies increases the acidity of blood. This condition, called ketosis, may result in coma if the alkalinity of blood is reduced considerably. Ketosis may occur in diabetes where the cells cannot utilize carbohydrates. The lower blood glucose levels may cause headaches in some individuals. To prevent these ketotic symptoms, it is recommended that the average person should consume at least 50 to 100g of carbohydrates per day.

4. Act as Flavour and Sweetners

A less important function of carbohydrates is to provide sweetness to foods. However, different sugars vary in sweetness. For example, fructose is almost twice as sweet as sucrose and sucrose is approximately 30% sweeter than glucose. Receptors located at the tip of the tongue bind to tiny bits of carbohydrates and send what humans perceive as a "sweet" signal to the brain.

Sweeteners are of two types i.e. nutritive or non-nutritive. Nutritive sweeteners include sucrose, glucose, fructose, high fructose corn syrup, and lactose. These types of sweeteners not only impart flavour to the food, but can also be metabolized for energy. In contrast, non-nutritive sweeteners provide no food energy and include saccharin, cyclamate, and aspartame.

5. Give Bulk to the Diet

Carbohydrates give bulk to the diet and play an important role in gastro-intestinal functions of mammals. They also add variety and flavour to the diet.

Deficiency of Carbohydrates

Carbohydrate deficiency diseases rarely occur, as carbohydrates are present in a wide variety of foods. However, one should not eliminate carbohydrates completely from the diet because the body then uses protein as an energy source.

Some foods contain only sugars. They do not contain any other nutrients. They provide empty kilocalories. Examples are carbonated drinks and table sugar. Too much sugar in the diet causes tooth decay and so many other problems.

Sources of Carbohydrates

Carbohydrates come from a wide array of foods. The best sources are cereals like rice, wheat, millets like ragi, maize, roots and tubers like potato, tapioca, sweet potato, yam and colocasia. The other sources

Carbohydrate	Source
Whole Grains	Brown rice, oatmeal, whole grain breads and crackers, whole grain ready-to-eat cereals like bran and shredded wheat
Starches (complex carbohydrates)	Cereal, potatoes, pasta, macaroni, rice, bread
Dietary Fibre	Whole grain cereals and breads, dried beans and peas, fruits and vegetables
Sugars (simple carbohydrates)	Fruit juices, fruits, sweetened cereals and baked goods, jam and syrup

are vegetables and fruits like banana, apple, plantain, pulses, sugar, jaggery and dried fruits.

Glycemic Index (GI)

Glycemic index measures how fast a food is likely to raise the blood sugar or is a ranking system for carbohydrates based on their immediate effect on blood glucose levels. It was invented by Dr. David J. Jenkins and his colleagues in 1981. In simple terms, a food with a higher glycemic value raises blood glucose faster and is less beneficial to blood-sugar control than a food which has a lower score.

The Glycemic Index Scale

The glycemic index consists of a scale from 1 to 100, indicating the rate at which 50 grams of carbohydrate in a particular food is absorbed into the bloodstream as blood-sugar. Glucose itself is used as the main reference point and is rated 100. Carbohydrates that break down rapidly during digestion have the highest glycemic indices. Such carbohydrates require less energy to be converted into glucose, which results in faster digestion and a quicker increase of blood glucose. Carbohydrates that break down slowly, releasing glucose gradually into the blood stream, have a low glycemic index. A lower glycemic response equates to a lower insulin demand, better long-term blood glucose control and a reduction in blood lipids.

High, Intermediate and Low Glycemic Index Foods

The glycemic index separates carbohydrates containing foods into three general categories: (1) High Glycemic Index Foods (GI 70+),that cause a rapid rise in blood-glucose levels. (2) Intermediate Glycemic Index Foods (GI 56–69) causing a medium rise in blood-glucose. (3) Low Glycemic Index Foods (GI 55 and below), causing a slower rise in blood-sugar.

Factors affecting Glycemic Index

The glycemic effect of foods depends on a number of factors such as:

- *Fiber content.* Fiber shields the starchy carbohydrates in food from the immediate and rapid attack by digestive enzymes. This slows the release of sugar molecules into the bloodstream.
- *Ripeness.* Ripe fruits and vegetables tend to have more sugar than unripe ones, and so tend to have a higher glycemic index.
- *Type of starch.* Starch comes in many different configurations. Some are easier to break into sugar molecules than others. The starch in potatoes, for example, is digested and absorbed into the bloodstream quickly.
- *Fat content and acid content.* The more fat or acid a food contains, the slower its carbohydrates are converted to sugar and absorbed into the bloodstream.
- *Physical form.* Finely ground grain is more rapidly digested, and so has a higher glycemic index, than more coarsely ground grain.

Uses of Glycemic Index—Diabetes and Weight Control

Although the glycemic index was invented originally to help diabetes patients manage their blood-sugar levels, dietitians and weight experts now use it as a tool to treat obesity, reduce cravings and appetite swings, and improve eating habits.

Glycemic Index							
Cereals		***Snacks***		***Pasta***		***Beans***	
All Bran	51	Chocolate bar	49	Macaroni	46	Baked	44
Bran Flakes	74	Corn chips	72	spagh, 5 min boiled	33	Black beans, boiled	30
Cornflakes	83	Doughnut	76	Vermicelli	35	Kidney, boiled	29
Grapenuts	67	Oatmeal cookie	57	***Soups/Vegetables***		Kidney, canned	52
Oatmeal	48	Pizza, cheese	60	Beets, canned	64	Lentils, green, brown	30
Puffed Wheat	67	Pizza Hut, supreme	33	Black bean soup	64	Red lentils, boiled	27
Fruit		Popcorn	55	Carrots, fresh, boil	49	Soy, boiled	16
Apple	38	Potato chips	56	Corn, sweet	56	***Breads***	
Apricots	57	Pretzels	83	French fries	75	Bagel, plain	72
Banana	56	Shortbread cookies	64	Green pea, soup	66	Hamburger bun	61
Cantaloupe	65	Strawberry jam	51	Green pea, frozen	47	Blueberry	59
Cherries	22	Vanilla wafers	77	Lima beans, frozen	32	Oat and raisin	54
Dates	103	***Crackers***		Peas, fresh, boil	48	Pizza, cheese	60
Grapefruit	25	Rice cakes	80	Split pea soup	66	Sourdough	54
Grapes	46	Rye	68	Tomato soup	38	Rye	64
Kiwi	52	Soda	72	Yam	54	Wheat	68
Mango	55	Cereal Grains		***Milk Products***		***Drinks/Juices***	
Orange	43	Barley	25	Chocolate	35	Apple juice	40

Glycemic Index *(Cont'd)*							
Papaya	58	Basmati white rice	58	Custard	43	Colas	65
Peach	42	Cornmeal	68	Ice cream	60	Grapefruit juice	48
Pear	58	Millet	71	Skim milk	32	Orange juice	46
Pineapple	66	*Sugars*		Soy milk	31	Pineapple juice	46
Plums	39	Fructose	22	Tofu frozen	115		
Prunes	15	Honey	62	Whole milk	30		
Raisins	64	Maltose	105	Yogurt, fruit	36		
Watermelon	72	Table sugar	64	Yogurt, plain	14		

Easy to Learn

- Strictly speaking, carbohydrates are not necessary for human nutrition because proteins can be converted to carbohydrates. The traditional diet of some cultures consists of very little carbohydrate, and these people remain relatively healthy. However, carbohydrates require less water to digest than proteins or fats and are the most common source of energy. Proteins and fat are vital building components for body tissue and cells, and thus it could be considered advisable not to deplete such resources by necessitating their use in energy production.
- All carbohydrates are ultimately converted into glucose. The use of the digestive enzyme amylase assists in better breakdown and absorption of carbohydrates.
- Very low carbohydrate diets can slow down brain and neural function because the nervous system especially relies on glucose. Glucose is the brain's preferred fuel.
- Foods high in carbohydrates are breads, pastas, potatos, bran and cereals are all high in carbohydrates.

- Carbohydrates are primarily an energy source as they convert to glucose, a cellular fuel. When not utilized for energy, can be stored in limited quantities as glycogen, a storage form of sugar. Carbohydrates cause release of insulin. If eaten in excess, are converted to fat, a storage form of energy, which can be stored in subcutaneous tissues, or can surround organs such as the liver or heart. Carbohydrates are one of the raw materials the liver needs to manufacture triglycerides, monounsaturated fats, and cholesterol.
- Complex carbohydrates (starches) include whole grains and starchy vegetables (dried beans, peas, squash, yams, etc.) Complex carbohydrates take longer to convert to glucose. They retain essential cofactors and micronutrients that are required for the carbohydrates to be fully utilized. Use of complex carbohydrates results in fewer insulin surges and less nutrient depletion. These are digested and absorbed through the small intestine and therefore provide more steady energy source for a longer period of time.
- Oat bran, a rich source of b-D-glucan, has been incorporated into many food products, particularly cereals, as a source of the soluble fibre that has been touted for cholesterol reduction.
- Simple carbohydrates are sugars (honey, syrups, candy, cookies, etc.) Fruits (especially juices) have metabolic effects similar to simple carbohydrates, even though not refined. Simple carbohydrates (sugars) cause greater insulin surges than complex carbohydrates. These are water soluble and readily absorbed into the body through the stomach, giving a burst of energy.
- If attempting to lose weight, it is most effective to limit intake of complex carbohydrates during the weight loss process. Other than fruits and fruit juices, it is advisable to totally stop all intakes of simple carbohydrates.
- If a person suffers from diabetes, or diabetes runs in your family, then it is also very wise to only use complex carbohydrates, again totally avoiding the simple carbohydrates. Be somewhat cautious with fruits and fruit juices.

- Fruits are best consumed one half hour before any other foods. Fruits will quickly enter into the small intestine for processing. Eating fruits in the midst of a large meal will keep the fruits in the stomach a long time, and allow the fruits to begin to ferment.
- The most effective method to loose weight is to keep complex carbohydrates to a minimum. Stop all simple carbohydrates. Do not eat any food after your evening meal.
- Then be sure to exercise every morning to get your metabolism in high gear so that a person burns off calories faster. Remember, the body has a built in starvation protector. One must turn the metabolism on, and place in high gear every morning by exercising, then consuming a sensible breakfast which could be the protein drink. If you go out for lunch during the work lunch break, avoid mixing proteins with carbohydrates, and especially avoid fast food establishments.

Review questions

1. What are carbohydrates? How can we classify them?
2. What are high and low Glycemic index carbohydrates?
3. Enlist various monosaccharides and disaccharides?
4. What is dietary fibre? How is it useful to us?
5. Write down the various functions and sources of carbohydrates.

2 Protein

Introduction

Protein (derived from greek word *protas* which means "of primary importance") is a complex, high-molecular-mass, organic compound that consists of amino acids. Proteins are among the most actively-studied molecules in biochemistry, and were discovered by Jöns Jakob Berzelius in 1838.These are essential for the structural and functional use of all living cells. Proteins also act as an important macronutrient in the human diet, supplying the body's needs for amino acids, the building blocks of proteins.

Composition of Proteins

Proteins perform different biological functions. These are class of bio-macromolecules, alongside polysaccharides, lipids, and nucleic acids, that make up the primary constituents of biological organisms and are essential polymers made up of a specific sequence of amino acids. Amino acids are known as the building blocks of protein and are linked together by peptide bonds.

There are Four Main Groups of Amino Acids

- Essential
- Non essential
- Conditionally essential
- Limiting amino acids

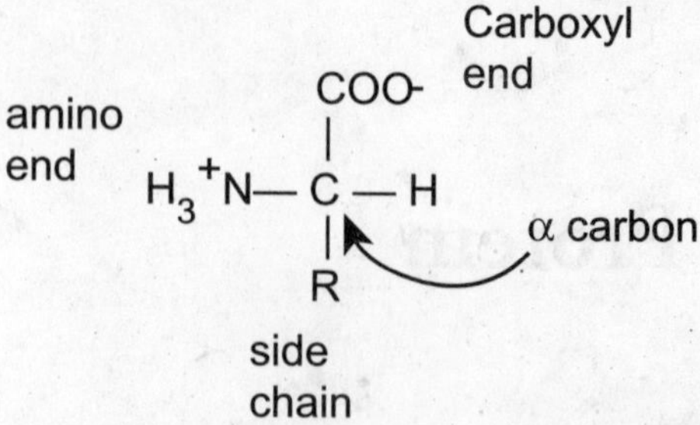

All amino acids have the same general formula

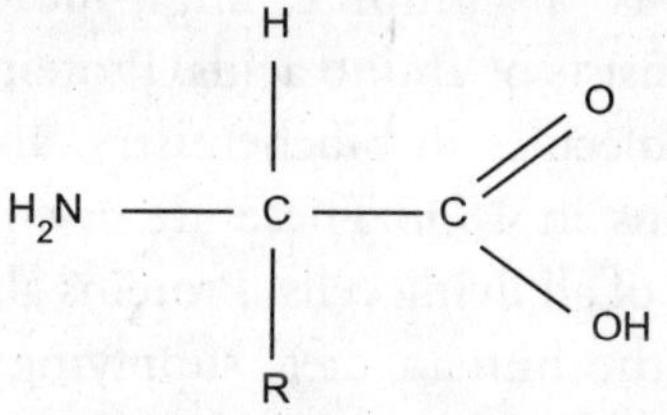

All amino acids have a similar chemical structure-each contains an amino group (H_2N), an acid group (COOH), a hydrogen atom (H), and a distinctive side group. All amino acids are attached to a central carbon atom (C).

1) Essential Amino Acids

Essential amino acids are also known as dispensable amino acids. Mammals cannot synthesize all 20 amino acids, so protein in the diet is necessary to acquire those that cannot be synthesized, known as essential amino acids. In humans, there are 10 amino acids, which the body cannot make and one should actually ingest them on a daily basis. Adults need 8 and children need 10 essential amino acids. The exact amount of dietary protein needed to satisfy these requirements for humans, known as Recommended Dietary Allowances (RDA) may vary widely depending on age, sex, level of physical activity, and medical condition. The eight essential amino acids include:

Isoleucine, Leucine, Lysine, Methionine, Phenylalanine, Threonine, Tryptophan and Valine. Some of these essential amino acids can be found in wheat, corn, beans, rice, beef and whey.

Arginine and Histidine are essential for infants as their body is not capable of synthesizing these amino acids.

2) Non-essential Amino Acids

Other name for non-essential amino acid is indispensable amino acid. The non-essential amino acids are those that can be produced within the human body. More than half of the amino acids are non-essential as the body can synthesize them. With the help of nitrogen to make amino group and carbohydrates and fat to make rest of the structure, the body makes any of the non-essential amino acid. All these processes occur in liver and known as transamination. These include: Alanine, Asparagine, Aspartic Acid, Cystine, Cysteine, Glutamic Acid, Glutamine, Glycine, Proline, Tyrosine, Arginine and Histidine. Cystine and Tyrosine are semi essential.

3) Conditionally Essential Amino Acids

Sometimes a non-essential amino acid becomes essential under special circumstances e.g. the body normally uses the essential amino acid phenylalanine to make tyrosine (a non-essential amino acid) but if the diet fails to supply enough phenylalanine or if the body cannot make the conversion for some reason, as happens in the inherited disease phenylketonuria, then tyrosine becomes conditionally essential. Similar is the case with Cysteine and Methionine. The Cysteine can be made from Methionine in human body.

4) Limiting Amino Acids

A limiting amino acid is an amino acid that is present in relatively small amounts but below the recommended essential amino acid requirements e.g. wheat has less amount of amino acid lysine. Lysine would therefore be called the limiting amino acid. A vegetarian would therefore have to cope up with lysine requirement by taking a supplement or by eating foods high in lysine, like soybeans and other legumes.

Classification of Proteins

Proteins are classified into two types:

Complete proteins: these proteins contain all the essential amino acids in sufficient quantity and ratio to supply the body's needs. They support life and maintain growth as well. These include proteins of animal origin, e.g. milk, meat, poultry and fish etc.

Incomplete proteins: these proteins are deficient in one or more of the essential amino acids and therefore do not support life on their own. Most of the plant proteins are incomplete proteins.

Protein Balance

The body's tissue proteins are constantly being broken down into amino acids in a process called catabolism and then resynthesized into tissue proteins as needed by the body, a process called anabolism.

To maintain nitrogen balance, a part of the amino acid that contains nitrogen may be removed by deamination then converted to ammonia (NH_3), excreted out as urea in the urine. The remaining non-nitrogen residue can be used to make carbohydrate or fat or reattached to make another amino acid, if necessary.

Nitrogen Balance

The body's nitrogen balance indicates how well its tissues are being maintained. The intake and use of dietary protein is measured by the amount of nitrogen intake in food protein and the amount of nitrogen excreted in the urine. For example 1 gm of urinary nitrogen results from 6.25 gm of protein. Thus if 1 gm of nitrogen is excreted in the urine for every 6.25 gm of protein consumed, the body is said to be in the nitrogen balance.

In states of malnutrition and illness, the balance may shift to either positive or negative.

Positive Nitrogen Balance

A positive nitrogen balance exists when the body takes in more nitrogen than it excretes, thus storing more nitrogen by building more tissues than it is losing by breaking down tissues.

This situation occurs normally during periods of rapid growth e.g. infancy, childhood, adolescence, pregnancy etc.

Negative Nitrogen Balance

A negative nitrogen balance occurs when the body takes in less nitrogen than it excretes. This means that the body has an inadequate protein intake and is losing nitrogen by breaking down more tissues than it is building up—an undesirable state of affairs. It may occur because

1) The calorie content of the diet is inadequate and therefore tissues are being broken down to supply energy.
2) The quality of the protein is poor or the amount fed is inadequate for the tissue replacement.
3) Injury, immobilization or disease are causing excessive breakdown of tissues.

Determination of Protein Quality

1) **Biological value:** BV is an index of protein quality that reflects the percentage of absorbed nitrogen from dietary protein actually retained by the body, measured under standard conditions.

$$\mathbf{BV} = \frac{\text{N retained}}{\text{N absorbed}} \times 100$$

2) **Net protein utilization:** NPU takes into account the relative digestibility of proteins.

   NPU = BV x digestibility

$$\mathbf{NPU} = \frac{\text{N retained}}{\text{Dietary N}} \times 100$$

3) **Protein efficiency ratio (PER):** It is defined as the change in body weight relative to the amount of protein eaten.

$$\text{PER} = \frac{\text{Weight gain in grams}}{\text{Dietary protein in grams}}$$

4) **Amino acid score:** it compares the content of essential amino acids in a protein or protein mixture with that found in a standard reference protein.

$$\textbf{Amino acid score} = \frac{\text{mg of amino acid per gram of test protein}}{\text{mg of amino acid per gram of reference protein}} \times 100$$

Functions of Protein

1) **Growth and maintenance:** The main function of protein is body building. They have many different biological functions and are classified according to their biological roles. Proteins are involved practically in every function performed by a cell, including regulation of cellular functions. They are the chief constituents of muscles, organs and endocrine glands.

2) Regulatory Functions in the Body

a) Enzymatic Proteins

Enzymes are proteinaceous in nature. They are the most varied and highly specialized proteins with catalytic activity. All the chemical reactions in the body are catalyzed by enzymes. There are thousands of different enymes, each capable of catalyzing a different kind of chemical reaction e.g. lipases help in fat digestion, amylases help in carbohydrate digestion etc. Digestive enzymes hydrolyze the polymers in food.

b) Transport Proteins

Transport Proteins play a very important role in the body. These proteins are involved in transporting other substances. For example, haemoglobin, the iron-containing protein of blood, transports oxygen from the lungs to other parts of the body. Other proteins transport molecules across cell membranes like lipoproteins transport triglycerides, cholesterol and fat soluble vitamins.

c) Structural Proteins

Structural proteins are very important for support. Collagen and elastin provide a fibrous framework in connective tissues, such as tendons and ligaments. Keratin is the protein of hair, horns, feathers, quills, and other skin appendages of animals. They are needed for mechanical support (skin and bones contain collagen-a fibrous protein).

d) Storage Proteins

These proteins store amino acids. Ovalbumin is the protein of egg white, used as an amino acid source for the developing embryo. Casein, the protein of milk, is the major source of amino acids for baby mammals. Plants store proteins in seeds and iron is stored in the liver as a complex with the protein ferritin.

e) Hormonal Proteins

Many hormones are made up of proteins. These hormonal proteins coordinate the bodily activities. Insulin and glucagon are the hormones secreted by the pancreas, which help to regulate the concentration of sugar in the blood.

f) Receptor Proteins

Receptor proteins are built into the membrane of a nerve cell and they detect chemical signals released by other nerve cells. They are involved in the cell's response to chemical stimuli.

g) Contractile Proteins

Actin and myosin are the contractile proteins. Actin and myosin are responsible for the movement of muscles. These proteins are very important in movement.

h) Defensive Proteins

Antibodies are the defensive proteins in the body. Antibody proteins are needed for immune protection. These proteins protect against diseases. Antibodies combat bacteria and viruses.

3) Protein as a source of Energy

1 gm of protein on oxidation produces 4 kcal of of energy.

Protein type	Example	Function
Enzymes	Amylase	Promotes the break-down of starch to the simple sugar glucose.
Structural proteins	Keratin, collagen	Hair, wool, nails, horns, hoofs, tendons, cartilage
Hormones	Insulin, glucagon	Regulates use of blood sugar
Contractile proteins	Actin, myosin	Contracting fibres in muscle
Storage proteins	Ferritin	Stores iron in spleen
Transport proteins	Haemoglobin serum	Carries oxygen in blood
	albumin	Carries fatty acids in blood
Immunological proteins	Antibodies	Rid the body of foreign proteins
Toxins	Neurotoxin	Cobra venom blocker of nerve functions

RDA of Protein

Protein is an important macronutrient in the human diet. The exact amount of dietary protein needed by the body varies widely. The recommended intake of protein is 0.8 to 1.2g per kilogram of the body weight depending on age, sex, level of physical activity, and medical condition. However, the athletes may need 1.0 to 2.0g protein per kilogram of body weight, which is referred to as the maximum protein intake: benefits ratio.

According to the recently updated Dietary Reference Intake guidelines, the recommended daily consumption of protein for adult men and women is: Women aged 19-70 need to consume 46g of protein per day. Men aged 19-70 need to consume 56g of protein per day. The difference is due to the fact that, in general, men's bodies have more muscle mass than those of women.

How much protein an individual needs in the daily diet is determined, in large part, by the overall energy intake, as well as by the body's need for nitrogen and essential amino acids. Physical activity and exertion as well as enhanced muscular mass increase the need for protein. Requirements are also greater during childhood for growth and development, during pregnancy or when breast-feeding in order to nourish the baby, or when the body needs to recover from malnutrition or trauma or after an operation. Because the body is continually breaking down protein from tissues, even adults who do not fall into the above categories need to include adequate protein in their diet every day. If an individual does not take in enough energy from the diet, the body will use protein from the muscle mass to meet its energy needs, and this can lead to muscle wasting over time.

Dietary Deficiency or Excess

As with any nutrient, moderation and balance are the key to health. Too much or two less dietary protein can be problematic in overall body function. Protein deficiency is usually rare. But it can occur in people who are dieting to lose weight, or in older adults who have a poor diet. A deficiency can also occur if the protein in the diet is incomplete and fails to supply all the essential amino acids. The following problems may arise due to the protein deficiency:

- Retarded growth in children.
- Worn out cells are not replaced. This prevents healing of wounds.
- Malfunction of various organs due to hormone/enzyme deficiency.
- Susceptibility to disease, due to lack of antibodies.
- In severe cases, as in underdeveloped countries, protein/calorie deficiency diseases such as kwashiorkor and marasmus may occur, particularly in children.

Protein Energy Malnutrition (PEM)

Two severe forms of PEM are kwashiorkor and marasmus. Kwashiorkor results from an acute deficiency of protein,whereas, marasmus results from a more chronic deficiency.

Kwashiorkor

It is an african word meaning a "diseaes of the displaced child" who is deprived of adequate nutrition. Occuring mostly in children between the ages of 1 and 3 years, when they are completely weaned (taken off the breast).

Manifestations and Signs of Kwashiorkor

- Oedema
- Moon face
- Growth failure
- Mental changes
- Hair and skin changes
- Infection
- Nutrient deficiency
- Water and electrolyte imbalance

Marasmus

Marasmus is more likely to affect individuals of all ages, suffering from inadequate food sources and is more common in children below the age of 2 years.

Manifestations and Signs of Marasmus

- Severe growth retardation
- Old man's or monkey's face
- Extreme emaciation
- Loose and hanging skin folds over arms and buttocks
- Absolute weakness

Protein deficiency can also cause fatigue, insulin resistance, hair loss, loss of hair pigment, loss of muscle mass, low body temperature, hormonal irregularities, as well as loss of skin elasticity. Severe protein deficiency, encountered only in times of famine, is fatal, due to the lack of material for the body to construct its own proteins.

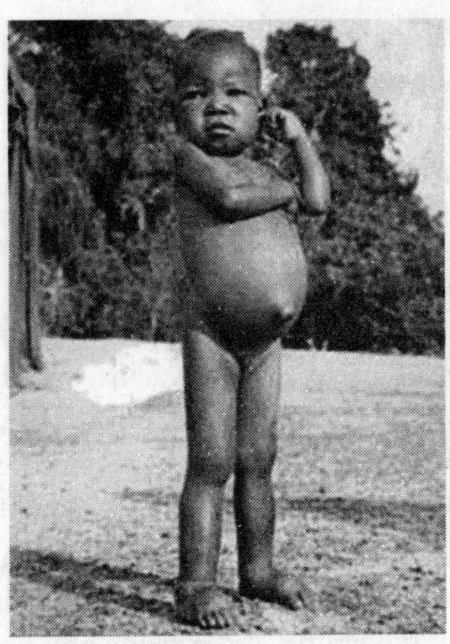

A case of Kwashiorkor

Excess Dietary Intake

The body has a finite need for protein, in other words, once a person has met the dietary protein needs, additional protein is deaminated (nitrogen is removed) and stored as fat or used as energy. The main problems with diets heavely laden with proteins are:

- These diets are usually high in saturated fats—a known risk factor for heart diseases.
- The kidneys have to work overtime to rid the body of excess nitrogen. Thus arises more chances of kidney problems.
- Excess protein increases calcium loses in the bones when dietary calcium is inadequate, which can lead to bone loss in the long-term.
- Loss of bone density, fragilty of bones is due to calcium and glutamine being leached from bone and muscle tissue to balance increased acid intake from diet (blood pH is maintained at around 7.4). This effect is not present if intake of alkaline minerals (from

fruits and vegetables, cereals are acidic as are proteins, fats are neutral) is high. In such cases, protein intake is anabolic to bone.

Sources of Protein

Animal foods are rich sources of this vital dietary element, while protein is also found in plant foods, such as grains and legumes, and in eggs and dairy products, such as milk and yogurt. In order to obtain the full range of essential amino acids, one should eat a variety of protein foods. Many people choose meat (beef, pork, and lamb) as their main source of protein, and eat it regularly through the week.

This is not necessarily the best approach. Animal meats commonly contain excess fat and lack other important vitamins and minerals, such as complex carbohydrates and dietary fiber. Plant foods, such as legumes, nuts, seeds, and grains, also provide protein. Soy products are particularly popular (e.g. tofu) but contain phytoestrogens, which can be harmful in excessive quantities. A combination of plant and animal proteins is recommended for a balanced diet. Although proteins are found in all foods, in less or more amounts, it is still well concentrated in foods such as legumes, nuts, and dairy products, the majority of which are protein choices for vegetarians.

Easy to Learn

- Proteins are best consumed away from any carbohydrates. This is especially true for those desiring weight loss.
- When protein foods are eaten, the protein (e.g. casein in milk and milk products, albumin in egg white, gluten in wheat and its products) is broken down into amino acids during the digestion. These amino acids are reassembled in the body in a specific order to form a variety of proteins e.g. collagen in connective tissues, myosin in muscles haemoglobin in R.B.C's etc. as required by the body.
- The proteins in the blood help hold salt and water inside the blood vessels so fluid does not leak out into the tissues. If albumin (the most abundant blood protein) gets too low, oedema occurs especially in the feet, ankles and lower legs.

Amino acids with hydrophobic side groups

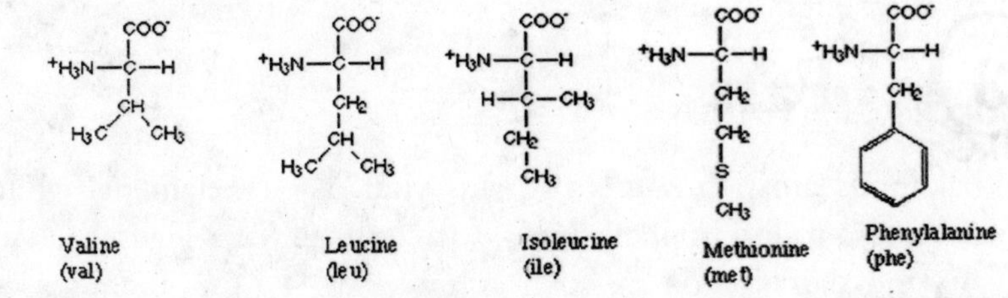

Valine (val)

Leucine (leu)

Isoleucine (ile)

Methionine (met)

Phenylalanine (phe)

Amino acids with hydrophilic side groups

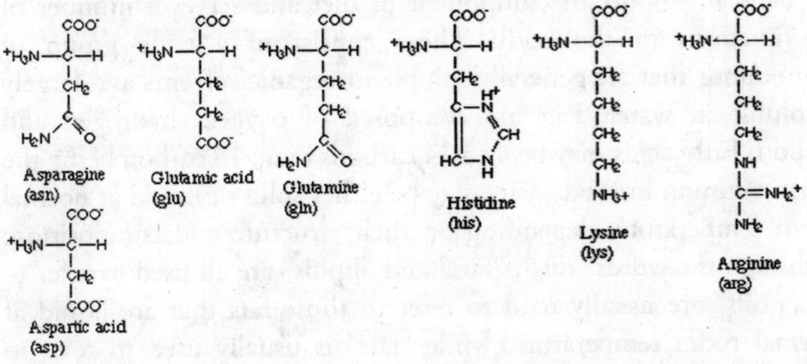

Asparagine (asn)

Glutamic acid (glu)

Glutamine (gln)

Histidine (his)

Lysine (lys)

Arginine (arg)

Aspartic acid (asp)

Amino acids that are in between

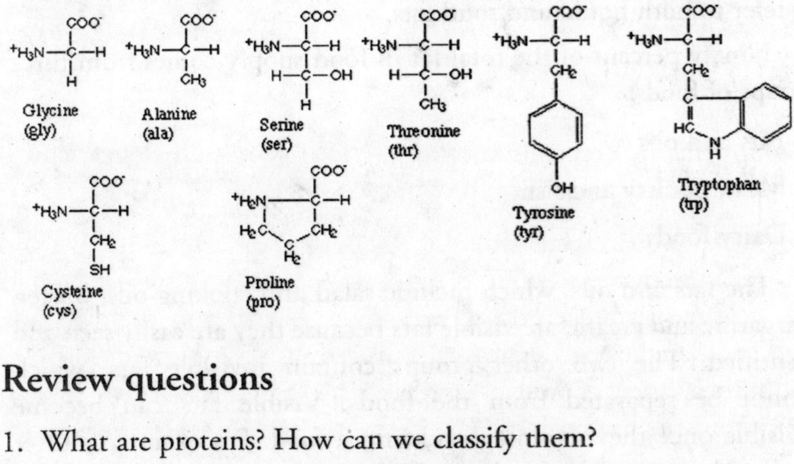

Glycine (gly)

Alanine (ala)

Serine (ser)

Threonine (thr)

Tyrosine (tyr)

Tryptophan (trp)

Cysteine (cys)

Proline (pro)

Review questions

1. What are proteins? How can we classify them?
2. What are the various methods for determining protein value?
3. Enlist various functions of proteins.
4. What is Kwashiorkor? Write down its symptoms.

3 Fats

Introduction

Fat is an important component of diet and serves a number of functions in the body. These consist of a wide group of compounds that are generally soluble in organic solvents and largely insoluble in water. Fats are composed of oxygen, hydrogen and carbon. Fatty acids may be 4 to 24 carbons long, 18 carbon being the most common in foods. Fats may be either solid or liquid at normal room temperature, depending on their structure and composition. Although the words "oils", "fats" and "lipids" are all used to refer to fats, "oils" are usually used to refer to those fats that are liquid at normal room temperature, while "fats" is usually used to refer to those fats that are solid at normal room temperature. "Lipids" is used to refer to both liquid and solid fats.

Ninety percent of the total fat in food supply comes from three groups of foods:

1) Fats and oils

2) Meat, poultry and fish

3) Dairy foods

The fats and oils, which include salad and cooking oils, butter, margarine and cream, are visible fats because they are easily seen and identified. The two other groups contain invisible fats, which cannot be separated from the foods. Visible fats can become invisible once they are integrated into a food. For example, butter on bread is a visible fat, but when used to make the bread, fat becomes invisible.

The difference between visible and invisible fat can also be described by looking at meat as an example. After trimming the outer layer of fat from the meat (the visible fat), 20 to 40 percent of its calories still come from fat distributed in the lean portion (the invisible fat). Other invisible fats are found in baked goods, nuts, peanut butter, processed meats and deep-fried foods such as potato chips.

Visible fats	Invisible fats
Oils, pickles, salad dressings margarine, butter etc.	Egg yolk, baked goods, whole milk, cream, cheese, nuts, oilseeds etc.

Chemical Structure

There are many different kinds of fats, but each kind is a variation on the same chemical structure. All fats consist of fatty acids (chains of carbon and hydrogen atoms, with an oxygen atom at one end and occasionally other molecules) bonded to a backbone structure, often glycerol (a "backbone" of carbon, hydrogen, and oxygen). Chemically, this is a triester of glycerol, being the molecule formed from the reaction of an acid and an alcohol.

Fatty acids may also differ in the number of hydrogen atoms that branch off the chain of carbon atoms. Each carbon atom is typically bonded to two hydrogen atoms. When a fatty acid has this typical arrangement, it is called "**saturated**", because the carbon atoms are saturated with hydrogen; meaning they are bonded to as many hydrogens as they possibly could be. In other fats, a carbon atom may instead bond to only one other hydrogen atom, and have a double bond to a neighboring carbon atom. This results in an "unsaturated" fatty acid. A fat containing only saturated fatty acids is itself called saturated. A fat containing at least one **unsaturated** fatty acid is called **monounsaturated**, and a fat containing more than one unsaturated fatty acid is called **polyunsaturated.**

Omega-3 and Omega-6 Fatty Acids

Omega-3 (ω3) and omega-6 (ω6) fatty acids are unsaturated "**Essential Fatty Acids**" (EFAs) that need to be included in the diet because the human metabolism cannot create them from other fatty acids. Since these fatty acids are polyunsaturated, the terms n-3 PUFAs and n-6 PUFAs are applied to omega-3 and omega-6 fatty acids, respectively. These fatty acids use the Greek alphabet (α, β, γ, ω) to identify the location of the double bonds. The "alpha" carbon is the carbon closest to the carboxyl group (carbon number 2), and the "omega" is the last carbon of the chain because omega is the last letter of the Greek alphabet. **Linoleic acid** is an omega-6 fatty acid because it has a double bond six carbons away from the "omega" carbon. Linoleic acid plays an important role in lowering cholesterol levels. **Alpha-linolenic acid** is an omega-3 fatty acid because it has a double bond three carbons away from the "omega" carbon. arachidonic acid is an omega-6 fatty acid.

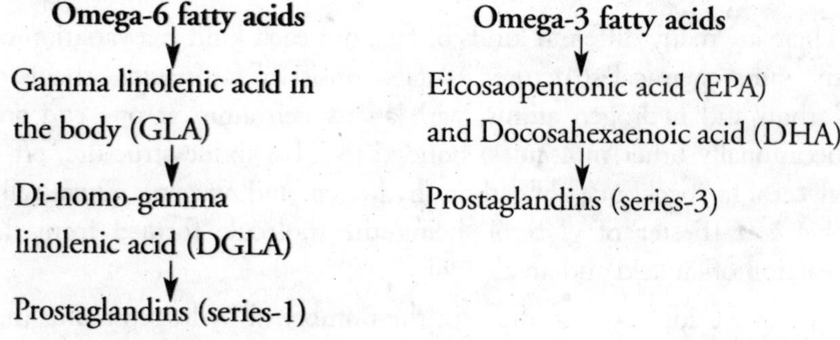

Prostaglandins are the hormone like substances, which are very short, lived and have important functions in the body. They help keep the blood thin, have anti-inflammatory influences on the joints, prevent fluid retention, help lower blood pressure and help insulin work efficiently.

Classification of Fats (Lipids)

Fats can be classified into three main groups:

a) Simple lipids

These are chemically made up of triglycerides. Triglycerides contain a glycerol base with three fatty acids. In a triglyceride the three molecules of fatty acids can be of the same acid or different acids.

Simple lipids are the neutral fats. These make up 98 to 99 per cent of food and body fats.

b) Compound Lipids

Compound lipids contain other radicals in addition to the three fatty acid radicals combined with one molecule of glycerol. Phospholipids are the compound lipids. Phospholipids are the compounds with a unique chemical structure that allows them to be soluble in both water and fat. The fatty acids make phospholipids soluble in fat, the phosphate group allows them to dissolve in water. Because of this reason the phospholipids are used as emulsifiers in food industry. Lecithin is the best known of phospholipids. Phospholipids have a backbone of glycerol with two fatty acids and a phosphate group and a molecule of choline occupy the third site.

c) Derived Lipids

This group includes fatty acids, alcohols, carotenoids and fat-soluble vitamins like vitamins A, D, E and K.

Functions of Fat

Fats are absolutely needed for life. They perform a number of important functions in the human body.

a) The Caloric Value of Fat

Fats provide a lot of energy in the form of calories. Calories are a measure of the heat produced by the utilization of foods in the body. Fats are composed of hydrogen, oxygen, and carbon, but fats don't have enough oxygen built into their structures to allow for breakdown. Oxygen has to be added into the mix from the oxygen in the blood. This process is called oxidation, and it gives rise to a great deal more caloric heat than is involved in the breakdown of carbohydrates or proteins, which do have sufficient oxygen. 1 gm of fat on oxidation produces 9 kcal of energy.

b) Body Fat as Storage of Energy

Body fat provides the most important reservoir of stored energy as adipose tissue. Adipose, or fatty tissue is the human body's means of storing metabolic energy over extended periods of time. Depending on current physiological conditions, adipocytes store fat derived from the diet and liver metabolism or degrades stored fat to supply fatty acids and glycerol to the circulation. These metabolic activities are regulated by several hormones (i.e., insulin, glucagon and epinephrine). In periods of low food availability or during a famine situation, a person lives on his/her stored body fat. This is how an individual obtains energy from the stored body fats. Fats are made up of glycerol combined with fatty acids. The glycerol is broken away from the fatty acids, and can then be converted into glucose for immediate use, and to glycogen for storage and later use. About 10 percent of the fat an individual eats is converted to sugars in a process called glyconeogensis.

c) **Fats as Transporters**

Another very important function of fat is transportation and use of vitamins A, D, E, K. Other fat soluble substances need fat to be digested, absorbed, and transported. Without fat in the diet, fat soluble vitamins would not be able to function and would result in severe problems like problems with eyesight, skin, nail formation, blood clotting, kidney function, bone growth and repair, reproductive functions, and cellular energy. Additionally, some of the fatty acids that make up fats are absolutely necessary for life. They are called essential fatty acids (or EFAs), because they must be eaten. Additionally fats slow stomach digestion and passage of foods through the intestinal path. This important fat function gives the body the necessary time to absorb the essential nutrients in the food.

d) Fat, in the form of structural body fat, provides important protection for the vital internal organs.

e) Fat is also necessary for the normal body development of children.

f) Fat is absolutely necessary for milk production in nursing mothers, and is required during pregnancy for the proper development of the child.

g) Fat is a fairly poor conductor of heat, body fat in the subcutaneous tissues (under the skin) acts as insulation, and tends to prevent loss of body heat.

h) Fats are required for brain structure.

i) Fat provides the makeup of the walls of cells, the cell membranes, which are required to allow the passage in and out of essential chemicals.

j) Fats are part of the structure of the skin.

k) Dietary fats stimulate the flow of bile, and the emptying of the gallbladder. Bile is important in the body's elimination of the waste products created by the normal breakdown of red blood cells. If the bile does not leave the gallbladder, gallstones may form.

l) Fats also provide the covering for nerves, and thereby allow nerves to carry the impulses necessary for different functions in the body.

Fats and Cholesterol

Cholesterol is a sterol. One should always "Eat a low-fat and a low-cholesterol diet." It is a simple way to lose weight and prevent cancer and heart disease.

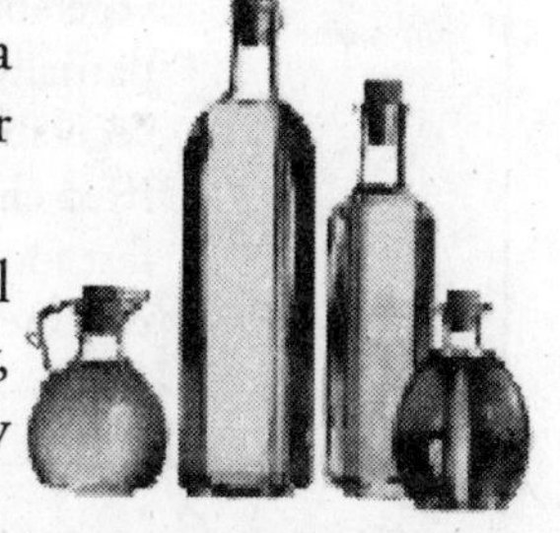

Detailed research shows that the total amount of fat in the diet, whether high or low, isn't really linked with disease. What really matters is the type of fat in the diet.

Bad fats, meaning saturated and trans fats, increase the risk for certain diseases while good fats, meaning monounsaturated and polyunsaturated fats, lower the risk. The key is to substitute good fats for bad fats.

Cholesterol in the bloodstream is also important. Although it is still important to limit the amount of cholesterol a person eats. High blood cholesterol levels greatly increase the risk for heart disease. But the average person makes about 75 percent of blood cholesterol in his or her liver, while only about 25 percent is absorbed from food. The biggest influence on blood cholesterol level is the mix of fats in the diet.

DIETARY FATS			
Type of Fat	**Main Source**	**State at Room Temperature**	**Effect on Cholesterol Levels**
Monounsaturated	Olives; olive oil, canola oil, peanut oil; cashews, almonds, and other nuts; avocados	Liquid	Lowers LDL; raises HDL
Polyunsaturated	Corn, soybean, safflower, and cottonseed oils; fish	Liquid	Lowers LDL; raises HDL
Saturated	Whole milk, butter, cheese, and ice cream; chocolate; coconuts, coconut milk, and coconut oil	Solid	Raises both LDL and HDL
Trans	Most margarines; vegetable shortening; partially hydrogenated vegetable oil; deep-fried chips; many fast foods; most commercial baked goods	Solid semi-solid	Raises LDL; lowers HDL

The Cholesterol—Heart Disease Connection

Cholesterol is a wax-like substance. The liver makes it and links it to carrier proteins called lipoproteins that let it dissolve in blood and be transported to all parts of the body.

Cholesterol plays essential roles, which are as follows:

- In the formation of cell membranes
- Some hormones
- And vitamin D

Too much cholesterol in the blood, though, can lead to problems. There is a strong link between high blood cholesterol levels and heart disease. Deposits of cholesterol can build up inside arteries. These deposits, called plaque, can narrow an artery enough to slow or block blood flow. This narrowing process, called atherosclerosis, commonly occurs in arteries that nourish the heart (the coronary arteries). When one or more sections of heart muscle fail to get enough blood, and thus the oxygen and nutrients they need, the result may be the chest pain known as angina. In addition, plaque can rupture, causing blood clots that may lead to heart attack, stroke, or sudden death. Fortunately, the buildup of cholesterol can be slowed, stopped, and even reversed.

Cholesterol-carrying lipoproteins play central roles in the development of atherosclerotic plaque and cardiovascular disease. The two main types of lipoproteins basically work in opposite directions.

Low-Density Lipoproteins (LDL)

LDL cholesterol is often referred to as the "bad" cholesterol. Because Low-density lipoproteins (LDL) carry cholesterol from the liver to the rest of the body. When there is too much LDL cholesterol in the blood, it can be deposited on the walls of the coronary arteries.

High-Density Lipoproteins (HDL)

High-density lipoproteins carry cholesterol from the blood back to the liver, which processes the cholesterol for elimination from the body. HDL makes it less likely that excess cholesterol in the blood will be deposited in the coronary arteries, which is why HDL cholesterol is often referred to as the "good" cholesterol.

In general, the higher the LDL and lower the HDL, the greater is the risk for atherosclerosis and heart diseases.

For adults age 20 years or over, the latest guidelines from the National Cholesterol Education Program recommend the following optimal levels:

- Total cholesterol less than 200 milligrams per deciliter (mg/dl)
- HDL cholesterol levels greater than 40 mg/dl
- LDL cholesterol levels less than 100 mg/dl

Dietary Fat, Dietary Cholesterol, and Blood Cholesterol Levels

One of the most important determinants of blood cholesterol level is fat in the diet—not total fat, but specific types of fat. Some fats are good for cholesterol levels and others are bad.

Cholesterol in Food

While it is well known that high blood cholesterol levels are associated with an increased risk for heart disease, scientific studies have shown that there is only a weak relationship between the amount of cholesterol a person consumes and their blood cholesterol levels or risk for heart disease. For some people with high cholesterol, reducing the amount of cholesterol in the diet has a small but helpful impact on blood cholesterol levels. For others, the amount of cholesterol eaten has little impact on the amount of cholesterol circulating in the blood.

Eggs

It has been found that moderate egg consumption—up to one a day—does not increase heart disease risk in healthy individuals. While it's true that egg yolks have a lot of cholesterol–and, therefore may slightly affect blood cholesterol levels—eggs also contain nutrients that may help lower the risk for heart disease, including proteins, vitamins B_{12} and D, riboflavin, and folate.

So, when eaten in moderation, eggs can be part of a healthy diet. People with diabetes should probably limit themselves to not more than two or three eggs a week, as for such individuals, an egg a day might increase the risk for heart disease. Similarly, people who have difficulty controlling their blood cholesterol must be cautious about eating egg yolks and choose foods made with egg whites instead.

Dietary Fats

a) The Bad Fats

Some fats are bad because they tend to worsen blood cholesterol levels.

Saturated Fats

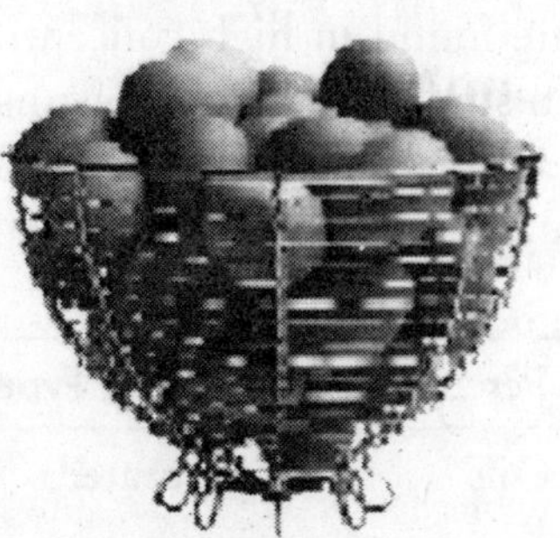

Saturated fats are mainly animal fats. They are found in meat, seafood, whole-milk dairy products (cheese, milk, and ice cream), poultry skin, and egg yolks. Some plant foods are also high in saturated fats, including coconut and coconut oil, palm oil, and palm kernel oil. Saturated fats raise total blood cholesterol levels more than dietary cholesterol because they tend to boost both good HDL and bad LDL cholesterol. The net effect is negative, meaning it's important to limit saturated fats.

Trans Fats

Trans fatty acids are fats produced by heating liquid vegetable oils in the presence of hydrogen. This process is known as hydrogenation. The more hydrogenated an oil is, the harder it will be at room temperature. Most of the trans fats in the diet are found in commercially prepared baked goods, margarines, snack foods, and processed foods. Commercially prepared fried foods, like French fries and onion rings, also contain a good deal of trans fat.

Trans fats are even worse for cholesterol levels than saturated fats because they raise bad LDL and lower good HDL. They also lead to inflammation, an over activity of the immune system that has been implicated in heart disease, stroke, diabetes, and other chronic conditions. While one should limit the intake of saturated fats, it is also important to eliminate trans fats from partially hydrogenated oils from the diet.

b) The Good Fats

Some fats are good because they can improve blood cholesterol levels.

Unsaturated Fats-Polyunsaturated and Monounsaturated

Unsaturated fats are found in products derived from plant sources, such as vegetable oils, nuts, and seeds. There are two main categories: polyunsaturated fats (which are found in high concentrations in sunflower, corn, and soybean oils) and monounsaturated fats (which are found in high concentrations in canola, peanut, and olive oils). In studies in which polyunsaturated and monounsaturated fats were eaten in place of carbohydrates, these good fats decreased LDL levels and increased HDL levels.

Percentage of Specific Types of Fat in Common Oils and Fats*

Oils	Saturated	Mono-unsaturated	Poly-unsaturated	Trans
Canola	7	58	29	0
Safflower	9	12	74	0
Sunflower	10	20	66	0
Corn	13	24	60	0
Olive	13	72	8	0
Soybean	16	44	37	0
Peanut	17	49	32	0
Palm	50	37	10	0
Coconut	87	6	2	0
Cooking Fats				
Shortening	22	29	29	18
Lard	39	44	11	1
Butter	60	26	5	5

Dietary Fats and Heart Disease

Most of the influence that fat intake has on heart disease is due to its effect on blood cholesterol levels. Ounce for ounce, trans fats are far worse than saturated fats when it comes to heart disease. It has been found that replacing only 30 calories (7 grams) of carbohydrates every day with 30 calories (4 grams) of trans fats nearly doubles the risk for heart disease. Saturated fats increased risk as well, but not nearly as much.

For the good fats, there is consistent evidence that high intake of either monounsaturated or polyunsaturated fat lowers the risk for heart disease.

Fish, an important source of the polyunsaturated fat known as omega-3 fatty acid. Eating fish may help prevent heart diseases. The omega-3 fats in fish appear to protect the heart against the development of erratic and potentially deadly cardiac rhythm disturbances. Nursing mothers and young children should include fish in their diets.

Dietary Fats and Cancer

Heart disease is not the only condition that has been linked with fat intake. Researchers once suspected an association between dietary fat and certain cancers like breast cancer, colon cancer, prostate cancer.

Easy to Learn

- Fats are broken down in the body to release glycerol and free fatty acids. Glycerol can be converted to glucose by the liver and thus used as a source of energy. Fatty acids are a good source of energy for many tissues, especially heart and skeletal muscle.
- Fat also serves as a useful buffer towards a host of diseases. When a particular substance, whether chemical or biotic reaches unsafe levels in the bloodstream, the body can effectively dilute or at least maintain equilibrium of the offending substances by storing it in new fat tissue. This helps to protect vital organs, until such time as the offending subtances can be metabolized and removed from the body by such means of excretion, urination, accidental or intentional bloodletting, sebum excretion, and hair growth.

- Use naturally occurring, unhydrogenated oil such as canola or olive oil when possible.
- Look for processed foods made with unhydrogenated oil rather than hydrogenated or saturated fat.
- Check labels of foods. Margarine may have high levels of trans fats due to hydrogenation. Choose margarines with liquid or pure vegetable oils as the first ingredient. Non-dairy whipped toppings and cream substitutes may also be high in saturated fats if made with coconut or palm oils. Look for those labeled "trans-fat free."
- Reduce intake of commercially prepared baked goods, snack foods, and processed foods, including fast foods. To be on the safe side, assume that all such products contain trans fats unless they are labeled otherwise.
- Limit the saturated fat in the diet.
- Eat commercially fried foods and commercial baked goods infrequently. Not only are these foods very high in fat, but the fat used is also likely to be hydrogenated, meaning a lot of TFA.
- Commercial shortening and deep-frying fats will continue to be made by hydrogenation and will contain TFA. That's just one more reason to eat fried fast food infrequently.
- Choose liquid vegetable oils.
- When foods containing hydrogenated or partially hydrogenated oils can't be avoided, choose products that list the hydrogenated oils near the end of the ingredient list.
- To avoid trans fats in restaurants, one strategy is to avoid deep-fried foods, since many restaurants continue to use partially hydrogenated oils. One may be able to help change this cooking practice by asking the chef, or manager if the establishment uses trans-free oils.
- Try to reduce visible fats in the diet.

- Bake, roast or broil foods instead of frying in fat.
- Use non-stick skillets without fat or use vegetable sprays.
- Remove any visible fat from meats and the skin from poultry before cooking.
- Add spices and herbs to vegetables instead of butter, sauces or gravies.
- Cool and refrigerate stews, broths and meat drippings and skim off fat before serving.
- Reducing invisible fat in the diet may be harder to do, but adopting the following practices will help.
- Choose lean cuts of meats instead of high-fat meats such as sausage, cold cuts, and spare ribs.
- Include fish, chicken and turkey in meals.
- Serve high-fat foods less often by substituting lower fat foods.
- Limit the intake of nuts, peanuts and peanut butter, which are all high in fat. Substitute skim or low-fat milk and their products (uncreamed or low-fat cottage cheese, low-fat yogurt, ice milk and mozzarella cheese) for whole milk and its products (cream, butter, ice cream and most cheeses).

Review Questions

1. What are fats? How can we classify them?
2. What are visible and invisible fats?
3. Enlist various saturated, monounsaturated and polyunsaturated fats.
4. What do you mean by high density and low density lipoproteins? How is it useful to us?
5. Write down the various functions and sources of fats.

Minerals

Introduction

Minerals are inorganic chemical elements that the body needs for healthy growth and metabolism. Minerals are defined as those elements which remain largely as ash when plants or animal tissues are burned. They are involved in making hormones and enzymes. Minerals are just as important as vitamins, and in fact work in conjunction with vitamins to perform many bodily functions. Minerals are often vital in the absorption, function and effectiveness of certain vitamins. If minerals are not present in the proper proportion, then vitamins are not sufficiently absorbed.

Many minerals are brought into the food chain of plants and animals through the soil, and the mineral content of soil varies from region to region, often leached out through poor farming methods. It is usually believed that the soil in many agricultural areas is so depleted of vital minerals that supplements are now necessary to ensure that the body gets an adequate supply of some of these essential elements.

General Functions of Mineral Elements

- Minerals are necessary for the formation of blood and bone, body fluids, cellular growth and healing, energy, muscle tone, and nerve function.
- All elements work together as a collective whole. If there is a shortage of just one mineral, the balance of the entire bodily

activity can be thrown away. A deficiency of one mineral may disrupt the entire chain of life, rendering other nutrients either useless or inefficient.

- All nutrients such as vitamins, proteins, enzymes, amino acids, carbohydrates, fats, sugars, etc., require minerals for their proper activity.
- The body must maintain an adequate mineral supply to maintain a "osmotic equilibrium." This state must be maintained for normal cell function. All bodily processes depend upon the action of minerals to work properly.
- Vitamins are required for every biochemical activity of the body but vitamins cannot function unless minerals are present.
- Minerals make enzyme functions possible. These combine with enzymes and complete the various works in the body like neutralization of the acid metabolic by-products of the cells and other toxic conditions within the body and prepares them for elimination.
- Hormonal secretion is dependent upon mineral stimulation.
- The acid-alkaline balance (pH) of tissue fluid is controlled by minerals.

Minerals have been divided into three main categories

- Macro Minerals
- Micro Minerals
- Trace Minerals

Macro Minerals

These minerals are required in large amounts at least 100 mg per day like calcium, phosphorus, sodium, chlorine and potassium.

Micro Minerals

These minerals are required in less amounts (generally less than 100 mg per day) like magnesium, manganese, iron, sulphur, boron etc.

Trace Minerals

These minerals are required in few micrograms including iodine, fluorine, zinc.

Macro minerals

Calcium–Ca

The body contains more calcium than any other mineral. Calcium and phosphorus account for 75 percent of total mineral elements in the body. Ninety nine per cent of the total calcium in the body is concentrated in the bones and teeth, the remainder is in the fluids and soft tissues. Calcium is an essential element for living organisms, being required for normal growth and development. It is absorbed from food through the walls of the intestine, and the process is helped by the presence of Vitamin D.

Main Functions

Calcium builds and maintains healthy bones and teeth, controls nerve and muscle excitability, controls conduction of nerve impulses, controls muscle contraction, aids blood clotting, controls cholesterol levels, helps in B_{12} absorption and reduces menstrual cramps. The need of calcium in the building of the skeleton is, of course, greater during the years of growth. However, the need does not end when full growth is attained. Once the bone is formed, it continues to change, with the processes of building new bone and maintaining the old. The normal behavior of heart muscles, nerves and the blood clotting processes all depend on the presence of calcium.

Building Bones and Teeth

Calcium and phosphorus are mainly present in bones and teeth. Calcium together with other mineral elements gives rigidity and permanence to bones and teeth. These characteristics make it possible for the bone to be the support of the body, providing the rigid structure for the muscle tissue attachment. Bone forms protective cavities for vital organs like the heart and lungs in the chest cavity and the brain in the cranial cavity. Bone will withstand almost as much weight as cast iron before breaking. It is itself light in weight.

Daily Allowances

Since the body does not absorb the entire calcium taken in the diet, extra allowances are always kept in mind while planning diets. The metabolic requirements for calcium recommended vary from 0.6gm to 1.0gm in different age groups. Pregnant, lactating women and growing children require more calcium.

Main Food Sources

Calcium is found in cheese, milk, mackerel, salmon and sardines, dried figs, tofu, low fat yogurt, sesame seeds, oats, millet, almonds, kelp, green leafy vegetables, parsley, pumpkin seeds and fortified cereals. It is estimated that the body normally only uses about 30 percent of the calcium present in the diet.

Main Deficiency Symptoms

Calcium deficiency is rare, but can occur when there is a lack of Vitamin D, or a problem with absorption through the intestinal walls. It can lead to conditions such as rickets, in children, and osteomalacia in adults. Rickets in childhood may encourage the development of osteoporosis in later life. A shortage of calcium will weaken bones, teeth, nails and hair, and may lead to the development of allergic reactions. Other deficiency symptoms include bone pain, muscle weakness and cramps, delayed healing of fractures, tetany (twitches and spasms), tooth decay, brittle nails, insomnia or nervousness, joint pain or arthritis, tooth decay, high blood pressure, fragile bones, menstrual cramps, eczema and rheumatoid arthritis etc. Repeated pregnancies coupled with inadequate dietary intake can also give rise to the deficiency of calcium.

Causes of Deficiency

- Low dietary intake
- Lack of vitamin D
- High intake of wheat bran, phosphates, animal fats
- The contraceptive pill
- Corticosteroid drugs
- Malabsorption due to low stomach acid
- Celiac disease
- Lactose intolerance
- Diuretic drugs
- Pregnancy
- Breast feeding

Excess (Hypercalcemia)

Excess of calcium and vitamin D in the diet causes severe disorders of calcium metabolism, which leads to hypercalcemia. Calcium in excess quantities can cause kidney damage—surplus calcium is deposited in the form of calculi (stones) in the kidney or bladder, or as tartar on the teeth. The body has mechanisms for regulating absorption and disposing of any excess by excreting it in the faeces, urine and sweat. Calcium competes with magnesium, and both minerals need to be present in the correct proportions for each to function. If there are high calcium levels in the blood, magnesium can help to reduce them, while calcium can help deal with potassium deficiencies. Many minerals and trace elements are interdependent. Hypercalcemia is treated by giving the patient a diet low in calcium and vitamin D.

Therapeutic Uses

Apart from maintaining the health of bones, teeth, hair and nails, calcium is required for maintaining the fluid balance in the body, sending nerve impulses and enabling muscles to contract. It is involved in the coagulation of blood, the functioning of the heart and the secretion of breast milk in nursing mothers. Calcium is taken on a daily basis for the bones and teeth, where it is stored, and constantly replenished. The levels of calcium in the blood are very carefully maintained, by two hormones, as small variations from the normal levels can cause cell damage and seizures.

Osteoporosis is a common problem, particularly for post-menopausal women, where calcium is withdrawn from the bones and not replaced. Therapeutic supplements of magnesium and calcium are used to treat osteoporosis, as well as other joint problems. To be assimilated into the bones, calcium requires the presence of both magnesium and silicon. The emphasis should always be on prevention rather than cure.

Magnesium–Mg

Magnesium is a metallic element, which is stored in the body's cells, primarily in bones and muscles. Dietary magnesium is absorbed into the blood stream through the intestine, but only about 30–40 percent of the available element is taken up. The percentage increases if less magnesium is consumed. The amount of magnesium available is diminished according to the quantities of calcium, phosphorus, protein, saturated fat and fibre in the diet. The amount of magnesium present in the body is less than that of calcium and phosphorus. A very small portion of it is bound to protein. A high calcium intake increases the requirement for magnesium as well. Excess is excreted from the kidneys and the unabsorbed magnesium from the diet is excreted in the faeces.

Main Functions

Magnesium is essential for the proper functioning of the body in many ways:

- It is required for nerves, muscles, the immune system and cellular function.
- Many different enzymes require magnesium in order to metabolise energy.

- It helps in strengthening of bones and teeth, promotes healthy muscles so helping them to relax.
- Beneficial for PMS, heart muscles and nervous system.
- It is involved as coenzymes for many functions in the body and essential for energy production.

Daily Allowances

The dietary intake of magnesium to maintain balance is around 350 mg/day. Magnesium content of foods is generally much higher than calcium.

Main Food Sources

Magnesium is found in green vegetables, whole meal flour, milk, eggs, fish, pulses, shellfish, nuts (especially peanuts), meat and cereals. A diet based on cereals, pulses and vegetables provides adequate magnesium to meet the daily needs.

Main Deficiency Symptoms

- Magnesium is essential for the muscles to function properly, and for proper communication between nerve cells. It is vital for cell division and for all reactions with phosphates.
- If cells become deficient in magnesium, the permeability of their walls changes, leading to the loss of both potassium and magnesium, these being replaced by sodium and calcium.
- In deficiency, muscles become weak, the person feels fatigued and may develop an irregular heartbeat.
- Deficiency of magnesium can lead to the development of kidney stones (due to excess calcium in the body).
- It also seems to be a factor in myocardial infarction.
- Deficiency in magnesium leads to a decrease in the efficiency of the autoimmune system.

- A shortage of magnesium can develop gradually, leading to a range of symptoms including anxiety, fatigue, muscle weakness, cramps, insomnia, restless legs and nausea.
- It may also be implicated in premenstrual tension.

Causes of Deficiency

Under normal conditions of health and food intake magnesium deficiency does not occur. A deficiency of it may result from malabsorption syndrome, chronic alcoholism, and toxemia of pregnancy or after intake of diuretics. Low dietary intake due to eating refined foods whose magnesium has been lost in the refining process and a lack of green leafy vegetables.

Excess

If taken in excess, it results in extreme thirst, excessive heat in the body and decrease in neuromuscular movements.

Therapeutic Uses

Helpful in depression, cardiovascular disease, PMS, muscle twitches and spasms. Large amounts of calcium in milk products, proteins, fats, oxalates (spinach, rhubarb) and phytate (wheat bran and bread), all deplete magnesium from the body. It works well with vitamin B1 and B6. Usually taken in conjunction with calcium, gives a good balance. Magnesium works combined with calcium in 3:2 (calcium: magnesium) ratio.

Sodium–Na

Sodium is present in many foods in the form of sodium chloride. About 50 percent of the total sodium present in the body is found in extracellular fluid. Bones, blood plasma and intracellular fluids account for the remaining sodium. Sodium can be easily interchanged between bones and the extra cellular fluid. Some of it is found deep down in dense long bones. The concentration of sodium in blood plasma is about 14 times more than that present in intracellular fluid.

The absorption of sodium chloride, which is an inorganic salt in the diet, occurs in the gastro-intestinal tract rapidly. Only small amount of sodium is excreted out in the faeces. The kidneys regulate the sodium level in the body. When the sodium intake is high, excretion is also high and vice-versa. If sodium is restricted in the diet, the excretion of sodium by the healthy kidney is absent and thus sodium is conserved completely in the body.

Sodium is also lost through perspiration, but this depends upon the concentration in the blood and the total volume of sweat. During the hot season the initial losses may be very high, because of that sodium depletion syndrome occurs. Salt and fluid intake should increase to make up for the loss of salt. Sodium loss in perspiration gets gradually reduced when the body gets acclimatized to the weather conditions. Sodium loss is more in Addison's disease (deficiency of adrenal hormone).

> Estrogen hormones favour sodium retention that accounts for oedema before the onset of menstruation and during pregnancy.

Main Functions

Sodium ions are the main ions in the fluid contained in the cells of the body. Their interaction with potassium ions is essential for survival and for the normal functioning of nerves and muscles. Sodium regulates the water balance in the body and maintains the acid-alkali balance. It is involved in the manufacture of adrenaline and amino acids.

Daily Allowances

8 to 10 gm of salt (sodium chloride) per day is sufficient for an average adult. A body adjusts to excess sodium intake. However, salt intake is restricted in the case of patients having a high blood pressure, cardiac failure and nephritis.

Main Food Sources

Sodium occurs naturally in most of the foods. The most common form of sodium is sodium chloride, which is table salt. Milk, beets, yeast extract, smoked fish, and celery also naturally contain sodium, as does drinking water, although the amount varies depending on the source. Sodium is also added to various food products. Some of these added forms are monosodium glutamate, sodium nitrite, sodium saccharin, baking soda (sodium bicarbonate), and sodium benzoate.

Main Deficiency Symptoms

Symptoms of sodium deficiency include intestinal gas, weight loss, poor memory, vomiting, low blood sugar, heart palpitations, and muscle weakness. Prolonged deficiency can lead to arthritis, rheumatism, and neuralgia (pain along a nerve pathway). But sodium deficiency is very rare because most foods contain some sodium.

Causes of Deficiency

Dehydration due to high temperatures, hard exercise or work, water intoxication, after sweating when thirst is satisfied with water containing no sodium. Sodium deficiency also frequently results during treatment with drugs called diuretics.

Excess (Hypernatraemia)

Too much sodium can raise the blood pressure, and make high blood pressure worse in people who already suffer from it. This can lead to heart and kidney problems. It can also cause migraines and lead to a condition called hypernatraemia, which is characterised by fluid retention and mental confusion, and may lead to seizures and even coma.

Therapeutic Uses

Salt replacement corrects the above conditions. A small fraction of the sodium combines with other minerals in the blood to prevent it from clogging. Sodium is found in the fluid surrounding the cells, helping to regulate the passage of nutrients, transmissions of nerve impulses, muscle tone and fluid volume. Salt is in abundance in processed foods. Over-consumption leads to fluid retention, loss of potassium, high blood pressure, oedema, weight gain, renal failure, and bronchial asthma.

Deficiency

Sodium deficiency is rare—but it can occur, either when sodium recycling is impaired by kidney problems, or when heavy sweating is caused by hot conditions or hard work. Symptoms include low blood pressure, dizziness, muscle weakness, respiratory problems, mild fever, weight loss and a general feeling of unwell ness.

Sodium Contributes to High Blood Pressure

- Increased salt intake causes more fluid to be retained in the blood vessels. This increased volume of blood makes the heart to work harder to pump blood to all the tissues in the body. Increasing the blood's volume within the enclosure of the circulatory system is one way that salt increases blood pressure.
- Salt elevates blood pressure through the action of the arterioles. Arterioles are blood vessels that dilate and constrict to regulate blood pressure and blood flow. By contracting under the influence of sodium, arterioles effectively increase the resistance to blood movement and lessen the volume of blood that is returned to the heart. This action also increases blood pressure.

The extent to which each person responds to high intake of salt is probably genetically determined. Some people are more susceptible to the effects of sodium than others. The sodium sensitivity appears to increase with age.

Individuals with the following characteristics may be at risk

- A family history of high blood pressure.
- Elevated blood pressure readings (normal is less than 120/80 mm/Hg).
- A high resting heart rate (given the level of physical fitness).

- A body mass index of 25 or higher. High blood pressure is a "silent" disease; it often has no symptoms. Everyone must monitor his/her blood pressure regularly.
- A diet high in potassium and calcium may help lower blood pressure.

Potassium–K

Ninety per cent of the total potassium present in the body is found in the cells. The remaining is distributed in the extra-cellular fluid. Plasma also contains small amounts of potassium. It is absorbed readily from the stomach and intestine. Potassium is also present in large amounts in the digestive juices. Excess potassium is excreted out from the kidneys. It is closely related to sodium, in that it often works with it, but to opposite effect. Potassium and sodium together control the electrical potential of the nervous system, allowing nerve signals to be transmitted and muscles to contract regularly.

Main Functions

- Potassium is required for the proper working of the nervous system, the muscles and the heart.
- It maintains the body's osmotic balance, and is required by several enzyme processes, including the metabolism of protein.
- The right balance of potassium is required to prevent cardiac arrhythmia.
- It helps in the secretion of insulin for blood sugar control, enables nutrients and waste products to enter and leave cells.
- It also stimulates peristalsis to encourage proper movement of food through the digestive tract.

Daily Allowances

The exact requirements of potassium are not known. A normal daily vegetarian diet provides this mineral in sufficient amount.

Main Food Sources

Potassium is found in most of the foods, particularly fresh fruits and vegetables (bananas, avocado, prunes, grapes, melon, dried peaches, tomato, potatoes etc.). Other sources include meat, milk, whole meal flour, coffee, tea and cereals. Coffee is one of our primary sources, as it contains about 45mg per cup.

Main Deficiency Symptoms

Potassium deficiency can lead to muscle weakness, fatigue, loss of appetite, thirst, low blood pressure, constipation and problems with the kidneys and nervous system. It affects the functioning of the heart. Potassium and magnesium deficiency both cause similar effects and tend to occur together. Potassium requires the presence of magnesium before it can be used by the body's cells. It is one of the most frequently prescribed mineral supplements. This is because levels are depleted by the use of diuretic tablets, which many people take.

Causes of Deficiency

Potassium is easily absorbed and excreted, unless there is some kidney malfunction. An excess of sodium may lead to an increased intake of potassium to maintain the correct water balance in the body. Therefore dietary excess is not usually a problem. However, diets high in fat, refined sugars and over—salted foods may lead quickly to a state of potassium deficiency. As humans age, the potassium levels drop substantially and this is one of the main reasons for the weakness and decline in strength of the elderly.

Excess

Generally speaking, the body excretes any excess potassium in the urine, but sometimes high potassium levels in the blood are caused by severe fluid loss—perhaps due to prolonged attacks of vomiting or diarrhoea. Kidney failure can also lead to an excess of potassium in the body. Symptoms of overdose include drowsiness, disorientation, weakness and cardiac arrhythmia, leading potentially to cardiac arrest.

Therapeutic Uses

Nausea, vomiting, diarrhoea, muscle weakness, irritability, swollen abdomen, confusion, mental apathy. Magnesium helps to hold potassium in cells.

Phosphorus–P

Phosphorus, chemical symbol P, is a non-metallic element, occurring naturally in the form of phosphate salts. Phosphorus is an important constituent in every body's tissue. The total amount constitutes about one per cent of the body weight. The amount of phosphorus in the body is exceeded only by calcium. In bones the proportion of calcium to phosphorus is about 2 to 1. In the body fluids and soft tissues the proportion of phosphorus is much higher than that of calcium.

Main Functions

Phosphorus is needed by the enzymes that metabolise fat, protein and glucose. It is essential for the processes by which the body produces and stores energy, and it helps in the formation of nucleic acids for cell division. It forms and maintains bone, teeth and is needed for milk secretion.

Daily allowances

The Indian Council of Medical Research has recommended a daily allowance of 1gm of phosphorus.

Main Food Sources

There is phosphorus in practically all foods, but particularly in high protein ones, such as meat, dairy, pulses as well as leafy green vegetables and most fruits. Carbonated soft drinks, red meat and junk food are loaded with phosphorus additives.

Main Deficiency Symptoms

Lack of phosphorus leads to weight loss, weakness, loss of bone density (it is required to make calcium phosphate, one of the main components of bone tissue), loss of appetite and stiff joints.

Anaemia and problems of the respiratory system and central nervous system are all associated with phosphorus deficiency. Phosphorus deficiency leads to calcification causing spurs and imbalance such as osteoporosis, loss of muscle control and strength, trembling, convulsion, high blood pressure, arteriosclerosis and heart disease. The deficiency of this element is very rare in humans.

Causes of Deficiency

Unlikely to be deficient in phosphorus.

Excess

Too much phosphorus in the diet prevents the proper absorption of calcium, zinc, iron and magnesium.

Therapeutic Uses

Eighty per cent of all the phosphorus in the body is contained in the bones. For the correct balance of calcium: magnesium: phosphorous, phosphorus plays a crucial role in determining how well calcium is absorbed, extracted and distributed in the body. This is because the two are stored together in the bone as a compound called calcium phosphate.

Boron, chromium, copper, iron, manganese, selenium, sulphur and zinc are the trace elements.

Boron

Boron helps absorb calcium into bones and keeps it there. There has been no RDA set for this trace element but many nutritional therapists suggest 3mg per day. There is usually no problem getting this amount from food and most people would absorb 2 to 5 mg daily.

Main Food Sources

Good food sources are fruits, especially apples, pears, peaches, grapes, dates, and raisins. Nuts and beans are also high in boron.

Chromium–Cr

Chromium is a metal that is found in small amounts throughout the environment (e.g. in the soil and in the air). It exists in several different "inorganic" forms, some of which can be toxic. It is a hard silvery trace element.

Main Functions

- Chromium is important in insulin metabolism. It is at the centre of a very small protein molecule that helps activate insulin receptors in the body's cells and because of that chromium helps insulin to work more effectively in the cells of the body.
- Chromium is important in the metabolism of fats and carbohydrates.
- Chromium stimulates fatty acid and cholesterol synthesis, which are important for brain function and other body processes. It is an activator of several enzymes, which are needed to drive numerous chemical reactions necessary to life.

Main Food Sources

The best source of chromium is brewer's yeast, but many people do not use brewer's yeast because it causes abdominal distention (a bloated feeling) and nausea. Other sources include whole grains, rye, oysters, green peppers, eggs, liver, mushroom, molasses and fruits like apple, orange and pineapple and peanuts etc.

Main Deficiency Symptoms

Anxiety, fatigue, glucose intolerance, adult-onset diabetes, excessive hot or cold sweats, dizziness or irritability, need for frequent meals, cold hands, excessive sleep or drowsiness during the day, excessive thirst, arteriosclerosis, improper glucose metabolism, hypoglycemia, diabetes, heart disease, decreased growth and improper fat metabolism.

Causes of Deficiency

High intakes of refined/processed foods.

Therapeutic Uses

Widespread deficiencies of chromium have been reported in developed countries. It corrects the imbalance in blood sugar levels and heart diseases.

Copper–Cu

Copper is widely distributed in nature. The adult human body contains between 80 to 150 milligrams of copper. The liver is the major location of stored copper, containing about 10 percent of the total-body content. The tissues of the body contain it in traces but the highest amount is found in the brain and liver. About 95 percent of copper present in blood plasma is found firmly bound in a protein complex, ceruloplasmin, and the remaining 5 percent loosely bound to another protein, albumen. Zinc and vitamin C supplements are strong antagonists of copper absorption. Most of the copper is excreted through the bile in faecal matter.

Main Functions

- Essential for life in small amounts. It is involved in many enzyme systems including one which protects us from free radicals and is needed to help iron carry out its functions of oxygen transfer to the cells.
- It helps in the manufacturing of a thyroid-stimulating hormone. And also assists in the formation of the insulation of the myelin sheath around the nerves.
- Helps to protect against heart disease and strokes.
- Good for bones and for the immune system.

Main Food Sources

Shellfish especially oysters, organ meats, cereals, dried fruit, almonds, beans and green leafy vegetables. Oestrogen-containing birth control pills may also elevate blood copper levels.

Even poor diets provide enough copper for human needs. Deficiency or excess of this element is very rare. Low levels of copper in the blood have been observed during malnutrition, in some kidney infections, sprue and in anemia. Toxicity of copper is well-known. Higher intake of copper can cause hepatitis, nerve disorders and malfunctioning of the kidneys. On the other hand a deficiency of copper makes the hair brittle.

Main Deficiency Symptoms

Anemia, hair problems, dry skin, general weakness, osteoporosis, arthritis, atherosclerosis, heart damage, skin sores, digestive problems and diarrhoea. Other symptoms include hardening of the arteries, high blood pressure, kidney disease, psychosis, early senility and other signs of early ageing.

Causes of Deficiency

High dose of zinc may induce copper deficiency, copper and zinc are strongly antagonistic so a deficiency in zinc can increase the absorption of copper. An excess of copper causes zinc loss. Vitamin C supplements are strong antagonists of copper absorption.

Therapeutic Uses

Copper deficiency is uncommon because of its abundant availability in drinking water via copper pipes. It cures rheumatoid arthritis. In large amounts it is considered toxic.

Iron–Fe

Iron is an important trace mineral that is found in every cell of the body, usually combined with protein. Iron is an essential mineral for humans because it is part of blood cells. It is the chief among the trace elements required for the body. In an adult it is approximately 3 to 5 g. It is widely distributed throughout the body. The major portion of it is found in the blood as haemoglobin. Muscle tissue contains about 3 per cent of iron as myoglobin and the rest is stored in the liver, spleen, kidney and bone marrow as ferritin, hemosiderin and siderophilin.

Main Functions

- Iron is part of haemoglobin in red blood cells. Iron transports oxygen and carbon dioxide to and from cells.

- It also makes up part of many proteins and enzymes in the body. And is vital for energy production.
- There is a small amount of iron in the plasma which is bound to a protein called transferin. In case of iron deficiency in the blood the level of plasma iron comes down and anaemia occurs.
- Iron is present in the muscle cells in two combinations, as myoglobin and as a constituent of haem enzymes. Myoglobin is a respiratory pigment present in the muscles of vertebrates and invertebrates. It is a compound of iron and protein. Myoglobin has the capacity of storing oxygen in the muscle for use in muscle contractions.
- The iron-containing enzymes in muscle make the oxidation of carbohydrates, fat and protein possible within the cell. These enzymes are the cytochromes, catalases and peroxidases. Each enzyme has the same functions, mainly bringing about the oxidative changes within the tissues.

Daily Allowances

The requirement of iron for the body is very small. A normal diet contains much more iron than what is required. Extra amounts have to be taken because less than 1/6 of the iron from the food is absorbed. Indian diets contain more of oxalates and phytates and less of proteins and vitamins, resulting in the poor absorption and utilization or iron.

Iron requirements recommended by ICMR per day are as follows:

Men	28mg
Women	30mg
Pregnant women	38mg
Lactating women	30mg
Children 1–9 years	12–25mg
Adolescent 13–15yrs	
Girls	28mg
Boys	43mg

Main Food Sources

Egg yolk, liver and meat are excellent sources of iron. Vegetarian sources of iron are cereals, millets, pulses, and green leafy vegetables. Of the cereal grains and millets, bajra and rice flakes are very good sources of iron but the rate of absorption of iron is less from all cereals. Other better sources of iron are jaggery, raisins, and dried dates.

On the other hand spices such as mustard, cumin seed, fenugreek, celery seeds and coriander contain liberal amounts of iron but they are consumed in small amounts. Milk of any source contains negligible amount of iron. When babies are on exclusive breast feed, the requirements of the body are met from the iron stores in the mother's body. These iron stores are adequate for a baby till 3 to 4 months of age.

Main Deficiency Symptoms

Anaemia, breathlessness, poor vision, insomnia, pale skin, sore tongue, fatigue or listlessness, loss of appetite or nausea, cramping, depression, palpitations and an under active thyroid gland.

Causes of Deficiency

Low dietary intake, heavy bleeding, menorrhagia and malabsorption due to lack of stomach acid.

Therapeutic Uses

Iron-deficiency anaemia, itching, impaired mental performance in the young and insomnia.

Haem and Non-haem Iron

Iron absorption depends in part on its source. Iron occurs in two forms in foods; as haem iron and non-haem iron.

Haem iron is found only in foods derived from the flesh of animals, such as meats, poultry and fish whereas, non-haem iron, is found in both plant-derived and animal derived foods.

Haem iron is derived from the haemoglobin and myoglobin found in meat and accounts for 10–25 percent of ingested iron. Prior to absorption the haem iron is cleaved from the globin. Absorption is influenced by body iron stores. The more deficient, the greater the absorption. Unlike non-haem iron, haem iron is relatively well absorbed and absorption is not affected by meal composition. Consumption of non-haem iron with haem iron increases non-haem iron absorption.

Factors enhancing non-haem iron absorption	**Factors hindering non-haem iron absorption**
Low body stores	Full body stores
Hydrochloric acid in the stomach	Reduction in stomach acid
Vitamin C	Oxalic acid (e.g. in Spinach)
Sugars	Phytic acid (in dietary fibre)
Haem iron	Calcium and phosphorus in milk

Non-haem iron is supplied by plant and dairy products. 2–20 percent of it is absorbed, the lower value being most typical. Non-haem iron consists mainly of iron salts, which are bound to foods and therefore must be hydrolysed or solubilised prior to absorption. **Stomach acid is essential for converting Fe^{3+} to Fe^{2+}.**

The average male tends not to have difficulty in maintaining his iron requirements, as many of them eat meat, poultry, and fish on a regular basis. However, because the iron requirements for women are much higher, because of menstruation, and because the requirement for energy (kcals) is less, and more women than men tend to be vegetarian, many women find it difficult obtaining enough iron. Pre-menopausal women need to choose iron-rich foods ideally at every meal, but at least every day. In general the bioavailability of iron in meats, fish, and poultry is high, in grains and legumes, intermediate and in most vegetables, especially those high in oxalates such as spinach, low.

Foods that contain vitamin C assist in the absorption of iron. A glass of orange juice will therefore aid the absorption of iron from a boiled egg. Meat, poultry and fish also aid the absorption of iron from other foods. For example, iron from baked beans will be improved if eaten with some meat, and the iron from bread would be enhanced by vitamin C in a slice of tomato on a sandwich.

Manganese–Mn

Manganese is an extremely important and valuable mineral, whose value for good health is just been recognized. Manganese is an essential trace mineral in human nutrition and is believed to be an essential trace mineral in animal nutrition, as well. Manganese is a metallic element. Its chemical symbol is Mn. It is required in small amounts in the diet. It is poorly absorbed from the small intestine. Manganese is transported by the blood as a loosely bound protein compound known as transmanganin. It is excreted as a constituent of bile but most of it is again re-absorbed and retained in the body. The amount excreted by urine is very small. This shows that the body can conserve the manganese very effectively.

Main Functions

- Manganese is needed for healthy skin, bone, and cartilage formation.
- It stimulates glycogen storage in the liver and also helps activate superoxide dismutase (SOD)—an important antioxidant enzyme.
- Acts as cofactor in over 20 enzyme systems involving growth.

Main Food Sources

Nuts, wheat germ, wheat bran, leafy green vegetables, beet, pineapple, black tea, and seeds are all good sources of manganese.

Main Deficiency Symptoms

In skeletal muscles, twitches, cramps, muscle tension, muscle soreness, including backaches, neck pain, tension headaches and jaw joint (or

TMJ) dysfunction. One may also experience chest tightness or a peculiar sensation that makes deep breathing little difficult. Symptoms involving impaired contraction of smooth muscles include constipation, urinary spasms, menstrual cramps, difficulty swallowing or a lump in the throat-especially provoked by eating sugar, photophobia, especially difficulty adjusting to oncoming bright headlights in the absence of eye disease, and loud noise sensitivity etc.

Causes of Deficiency

High intakes of refined/processed foods, long-term zinc deficiency, rarely due to excess copper intake, alcohol, malabsorption, and certain antibiotics.

Therapeutic Uses

Manganese plays a role in bone metabolism, it has been suggested as a treatment for **osteoporosis**, a condition in which bone mass deteriorates with age. Manganese may help control symptoms of dysmenorrhea (menstrual pain). Manganese has also been suggested for the treatment of muscle strains and sprains. People with epilepsy or diabetes have lower-than-normal levels of manganese in their blood.

Selenium–Se

The essential trace mineral, selenium, is of fundamental importance to human health. Selenium has additional important health effects particularly in relation to the immune response and cancer prevention. Deficiency has been linked to adverse mood states. An elevated selenium intake may be associated with reduced cancer risk.

Main Functions

- As a constituent of selenoproteins, selenium has structural and enzyme roles.
- Best-known as an antioxidant and catalyst for the production of active thyroid hormone.
- Selenium is needed for the proper functioning of the immune system.

- Appears to be a key nutrient in counteracting the development of virulence and inhibiting HIV progression to AIDS.
- It is required for sperm motility and supports male reproduction.
- Reduces the risk of miscarriage.
- Protects the body against toxic metabolites and cancer as an antioxidant and cofactor of glutathione peroxides.
- Protects against toxic minerals.
- Maintenance of normal liver function.
- Production of prostaglandins.
- Maintains the health of eyes, hair and skin.
- Acts as anti-inflammatory agent.
- Maintains the health of the heart.
- Potentate's action of vitamin E and helps produce coenzyme Q.

Main Food Sources

Plant foods are the major dietary sources of selenium in most countries throughout the world. The content of selenium in food depends on the selenium content of the soil where plants are grown or animals are raised.

Selenium also can be found in some meats and seafood. Animals that eat grains or plants that were grown in selenium-rich soil have higher levels of selenium in their muscle. Some nuts are also sources of selenium. Selenium occurs in foods such as corn, wheat, and soybean.

Main Deficiency Symptoms

- Cataracts
- Impaired growth
- Heart disease
- Reduced immunity and resistance to infections
- Inflammation of the muscles

- Reduced fertility in men
- Cancerous changes
- The reduced ability to detoxify

Causes of Deficiency

High intake of refined/processed foods and/or high intake of foods grown on selenium-deficient soil.

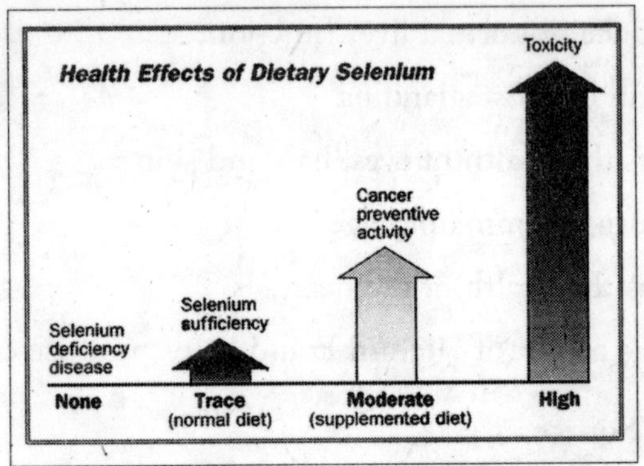

Sulphur–S

Sulphur is an essential element in living organisms, occurring in the amino acids cysteine and methionine, and therefore in many proteins. It is also a constituent of various cell metabolites, e.g., coenzyme A. Sulphur is absorbed by plants from soil.

Main Functions

Joint protection and repair, antioxidant/free radical scavenger, protection and strengthening of skin, hair and nail tissue, detoxification, heavy metal removal and general connective tissue repair. Helps in maintaining the oxygen balance necessary for proper brain function.

Main Food Sources

Egg, onions, garlic, seafood, milk, cabbage, lean beef, dried beans.

Main Deficiency Symptoms

Joint aches and pains, frequent infections, poor nails, hair, and skin, back pain.

Causes of Deficiency

Insufficient intake in the diet, stress, excessive exercise.

Therapeutic Uses

Rheumatoid arthritis, after strain or injury, back pain, joint pain, reducing inflammation caused by damage or overuse, improves circulation. Sulphur acts as a very powerful antioxidant. Works well with B - complex group of vitamins, forms part of the tissue, helps in building amino acids, known as the sulphur—containing amino acids.

Zinc–Zn

It is found in traces in all body tissues, the content being 1.2 grams of it in adults. The highest concentration of it occurs in the liver, pancreas, kidneys and brain. It is also present in red blood cells and blood serum. Zinc is poorly absorbed from the intestine and most of it is excreted in the faeces. A small amount of zinc is also excreted through urine. A high calcium and phytate intake interferes with the absorption of zinc.

Main Functions

Numerous aspects of cellular metabolism are zinc-dependent. Zinc plays an important role in growth and development, the immune response, neurological function, and reproduction. On the cellular level, the function of zinc can be divided into three categories: 1) catalytic, 2) structural, and 3) regulatory

1) Catalytic

Nearly 100 different enzymes depend on zinc for their ability to catalyze vital chemical reactions. Zinc-dependent enzymes can be found in all known classes of enzymes.

2) Structural

Zinc plays an important role in the structure of proteins and cell membranes. Loss of zinc from biological membranes increases their susceptibility to oxidative damage and impairs their function.

3) Regulatory

Zinc plays an important role in hormone release and nerve impulse transmission.

Zinc is also essential for bone growth, sexual development, energy production and maintenance of blood sugar levels (as it is needed for insulin production). It is needed to use vitamin B_6 and vitamin A efficiently, and carries carbon dioxide from the cells to lungs. It maintains acid-alkaline balance in the body and is an essential mineral in maintaining the health of the prostate, ovaries and testes. Zinc boosts the immune system.

Main Food Sources

Zinc is present in most foods both of vegetable and of animal origin, but the richest sources tend to be protein-rich foods such as meat, seafoods and eggs. In developing countries, however, where most people consume relatively small amounts of these foods, most zinc comes from cereal grains and legumes.

Main Deficiency Symptoms

- Poor appetite
- Lethargy
- Abnormal sight, smell or taste
- Low resistance to infection
- Hyperactivity in children
- Low fertility
- Growth failure (dwarfism) and hypogonadism are also associated with zinc deficiency.

Causes of Deficiency

Kidney disease, alcoholism, oestrogen also affects zinc levels, the contraceptive pill causes a drop in zinc, as does the high level of natural oestrogen in the body before a period, frequent sexual intercourse in men, high intake of refined/processed foods.

Therapeutic Uses

Frequent infections, stretch marks, acne or greasy skin, poor appetite, tendency to depression, low fertility, loss of menstruation. Phytates and oxalates prevent zinc from being absorbed. Care must be taken as zinc and copper are highly antagonistic - a high intake of zinc may induce a copper deficiency. Many zinc supplements are in the market.

Zinc Toxicity

- Individuals may be exposed to high intakes of zinc, either through supplemental zinc or by contact with environmental zinc.
- Overt toxicity symptoms, such as nausea, vomiting, epigastric pain, diarrhea and lethargy may occur with acute high intakes.
- Approximately 200 to 400 mg zinc is known to produce immediate vomiting in adults.
- Chronic overdosage of zinc, in the range of 100 to 300 mg zinc per day for adults may induce copper deficiency and alterations in the immune response.

Fluorine

Fluorine is a trace element that is found in a great variety of foods, in very small amounts. It is never found free in nature. Traces of fluorine are present in bones, teeth, thyroid gland and skin. It protects teeth from decay.

Main Functions

Fluorine is a mineral found mainly in the teeth and skeleton. Traces of fluorine in the teeth help to protect them against decay. Fluorides consumed during childhood become a part of the dental enamel and make it more resistant to the weak organic acids formed from foods that adhere to or get stuck between the teeth. This strengthening greatly reduces the chances of decay or caries developing in the teeth. Some studies have suggested that fluoride may also help strengthen bones, particularly later in life, and may thus inhibit the development of osteoporosis.

Daily Allowances

Fluoride is required in small amounts only. A small amount, 1ppm, is considered enough for normal healthy teeth. Soft water has little or no fluoride, while in hard water the fluoride content may be as high as 10 ppm. The average adult man may ingest about one milligram of fluorine daily from drinking water that contains one part per million (1ppm). In addition the average diet may provide 0.25 to 0.35mg of fluorine.

Main Food Sources

The main source of fluorine for most human beings is the drinking water. If the water has fluorine content of about one part per million (1 ppm), then it will supply adequate fluorine for the teeth. However, many water supplies contain much less than this amount. Fluorine is present in bones, consequently small fish that are consumed whole, are a good source. Tea has high fluorine content.

Deficiency

Fluorine is often known as a two-edged sword. If the fluoride content of drinking-water in any locality is below 0.5 ppm, dental caries will probably be much more prevalent than, where the concentration is higher.

The recommended level of fluoride in water is between 0.8 and 1.2 ppm. In some countries or localities where the content of fluorine in the water is less than 1 ppm, it has now become the practice to add fluoride to the water supply. This practice is strongly recommended, but it is only practicable for large piped-water supplies; in some developing countries where most people do not have piped water, it is not feasible. The addition of fluoride to toothpaste also helps reduce dental caries. Fluorine does not totally prevent dental caries, but it can reduce the incidence by 60 to 70 percent.

Excess

An excessively high intake of fluoride causes a condition known as dental fluorosis, in which the teeth become mottled. It is usually caused by consuming excessive fluoride in water supplies that have high fluoride levels. Very high fluorine intakes also cause bone changes with sclerosis (added bone density). Skeletal fluorosis can cause severe pain and serious bone abnormalities.

Iodine

Iodine is required for growth and survival. It is widespread in the environment, but is chiefly derived from the ocean and the soil. About one-third of the iodine present in adults occurs in the thyroid gland i.e. about 25 to 50 mg.

The degree of absorption of iodine in the body depends upon the level of the thyroid hormone circulating in the blood. The blood transports iodine as free iodine and as protein bound iodine (PBI).

Main Functions

- It is a constituent of the thyroid gland, which controls the rate of energy utilized in the body or the BMR.
- Iodine is essential for synthesis of the thyroid hormone, thyroxine.
- Thyroxine regulates the rate of oxidation within the cells thereby stimulating physical and mental growth, functioning of nerve and muscle tissue, circulation of blood and metabolism of all nutrients.

Daily Allowances

A teaspoon of iodine is all a person requires in a lifetime. However, the thyroid gland does not have the capacity to store this amount, so small amounts of iodine must be consumed regularly in the diet. The World Health Organization recommends the following daily intake for optimal iodine nutrition:

WHO daily intake: optimal iodine nutrition

Population sub-group	Amount
Adults	150 μg/day
Pregnancy and Lactation	200 μg/day
Children (6–12 years)	120 μg/day
Infants (0–5 years)	90 μg/day

Main Food Sources

The richest natural food sources of iodine are seafood and seaweeds (such as kelp and nori), because the ocean is a rich reservoir of iodine. The iodine levels in foods of animal origin (eggs, meat and dairy products) are higher than in most foods of plant origin, and they may have been further enriched by the use of iodine-supplemented animal feed. Iodine is generally supplied by food and water, provided the soil contains it.

In hilly areas where there is deficiency of iodine in food and drinking water, iodisation of salt is the only technique available to correct this deficiency in order to prevent endemic goiter. Sodium or Potassium iodide is used for iodization. In areas where salt iodization is not possible, another method is employed in which the iodised oil is injected into the muscles.

Deficiency of Iodine

A diet lacking in iodine is associated with a wide spectrum of adverse health effects collectively known as Iodine Deficiency Disorders (IDD's). IDD's can affect people of all ages, but most severely affects the foetus in the womb or in the period soon after birth. Iodine deficiency has the greatest impact during pregnancy, due to its devastating effects on the baby's developing brain and also on physical growth. In the worst cases of severe iodine deficiency, a child may born with cretinism, a condition characterised by severe mental retardation, growth stunting, apathy, impaired movement and speech or hearing.

Deficiency of Iodine causes goitre, which is characterized by the swelling of the thyroid gland. The reduced secretion of the thyroid gland leads to several other problems in the body.

Hypothyroidism

Endemic goiter, the iodine deficiency disease, occurs in certain parts of the world where the soil has low iodine content. As a result the food and water also become deficient in iodine in these areas. Endemic goitre is a public health problem in India, especially in the sub-Himalayan areas.

Hyperthyroidism

Due to the over-activity of thyroid gland there is excessive oxidation of food. The individual with a hyperactive thyroid will be lean, restless, perpetually hungry, having bulging eyes (exophthalmic goitre). The presence of a natural inhibitor of thyroxine in cabbage, turnips, mustard and rapeseeds help to over come hyperthyroidism.

Mineral	Functions	Sources	Signs of Deficiencies	Signs of Excessive Intake
Macro Minerals:				
Calcium (Ca)	Key constituent of bones and teeth. Essential for vital metabolic processes such as nerve function, muscle contraction, and blood clotting.	Dairy Products	Deficiency (or insufficient uptake) may lead to: Osteomalacia, Osteoporosis, Rickets, Tetany.	Formation of "stones" in the body, especially the Gall Bladder and the Kidneys.
Iron (Fe)	Essential for transfer of oxygen between tissues in the body.	Blood (e.g. "Black Pudding"); Eggs; Green (leafy) vegetables; Fortified foods (e.g. cereals, white flour); Liver.	Deficiency may lead to: Peas; Whole grains. Anaemia, Increased susceptibility to infections.	Long-term excessive intake of iron can lead to: Haemochromatosis or Meat; Nuts; Offal; Haemosiderosis (involving organ damage), and both of which are rare; Insufficient calcium and magnesium in the body (because these minerals compete with each other for absorption). Increased susceptibility to infectious diseases.

Mineral	Functions	Sources	Signs of Deficiencies	Signs of Excessive Intake
Macro Minerals:				
Magnesium (Mg)	Essential for healthy bones; Functioning of muscle & nervous tissue; Needed for functioning of approx. 90 enzymes.	Eggs; Green leafy vegetables; Fish (esp. shellfish); Milk (and dairy products); Nuts; Wholemeal flour.	Deficiency can occur gradually, leading to: Anxiety; Fatigue; Insomnia; Muscular problems; Nausea; Premenstrual problems. The extreme cases of deficiency may be associated with arrhythmia.	Unusual.
Phosphorous (P)	Constituent of bone tissue; Forms compunds needed for energy conversion reactions (e.g. ATP).	Dairy products; fruits (most fruits); Meat; Pulse; Vegetables	Insufficient phosphorous may lead to:Anaemia; Demineralization of bones Nerve disorders; Respiratory problems; Weakness; Weight Loss	Excess phosphorous can interfere with the body's absorption of: calcium, iron, magnesium, and zinc.
Potassium (K)	Main ion of intracellular fluid; Necessary to maintain electrical potentials of the nervous system and so functio-ing of muscle and nerve tissues.	Cereals Coffee; Fresh Fruits; Meat; Salt-subsitutes; Whole-grain flour.	Insufficient potassium in the body may lead to: General muscle paralysis; Metabolic disturbances.	Excessive amounts in the body (whether due to intake or other causes) may lead to:Arrhythmia, and ultimately cardiac arrest ("heart attack") Metabolic disturbances.

Mineral	Functions	Sources	Signs of Deficiencies	Signs of Excessive Intake
Macro Minerals:				
Sodium (Na)	Controls the volume of extra cellular fluid in the body; Maintains the acid-alkali (pH) balance in the body. Necessary to maintain electrical potentials of the nervous system and so functioning of muscle and nerve tissues.	Processed bakery products; Processed foods generally (incl. tinned and cured products); Table Salt.	Insufficient sodium in the body may lead to Low blood pressure. General muscle weakness/ paralysis; Mild Fever; Respiratory problems.	Excessive amounts in the body (whether due to intake or other causes) may lead to: Hypernatraemia; De-hydration (especially in babies); Possible long-term effects may include hypertension.
Macro Minerals:				
Chromium (Cr)	Involved in the functioning of skeletal muscle.	Cereals; Cheese; Fresh fruit; Meat; Nuts; Wholemeal flour	Deficiency may lead to: Confusion; Depression; Irritability; Weakness.	
Copper (Cu)	Part of the enzyme copper-zince superoxide dismutase (CuZn SOD); Also present in other enzymes, including	Cocoa; Liver; Kidney; Oysters; Peas; Raisins.	Insufficient copper has been associated with: changes in hair colour and texture, and hair loss; disturbances to the	

Mineral	Functions	Sources	Signs of Deficiencies	Sign of Excessive Intake
Macro Minerals:				
	cytochrome oxidase, ascorbic acid oxidase, and tyrosinases; Found in the red blood cells, and in blood plasma.		nervous system; bone diseases. Serious deficiency is rare but can lead to: Menke's syndrome.	
Manganese (Mn)	Antioxidant properties; Fertility; Formation of strong healthy bones, nerves, and muscles; Forms part of the enzyme copper-zince superoxide dismutase (CuZn SOD) system;	Avocados; Nuts; Pulses; Tea; Vegetables; Whole -grain cereals.	Deficiencies are unusual but may lead to: Bone deformities; Rashes & skin conditions; Reduced hair growth; Retarded growth (in children).	Excessive intake has been associated with brain conditions such as symtoms similar to those resulting from Parkinson's disease
Sulphur (S)	Healing build-up of toxic substances in the body; Structural health of the body (sulphur is a part of many amino acids incl. cysteine and methionine), Healthy skin, nails and hair.	Beans; Beef; Cruciferous vegetables (e.g broccoli), Dairy produce; Meat	Deficiency of sulphur is unusual.	

Mineral	Functions	Sources	Signs of Deficiencies	Signs of Excessive Intake
Macro Minerals:				
Zinc (Zn)	Needed for: Functioning of many (over 200) enzymes, Strong immune system.	Dairy produce, Egg yolk, Liver, Red meat, Seafood, Whole-grain flour.	Deficiency is rare but may lead to: Lesions on the skin, oesophagus and cornea. Retarded growth (of children); Susceptibility to infection.	Excessive intake is not a common problem but espe cially if zinc supplements are taken over an extended period of time, can reduce the absorption of Copper (so Copper supplements may also be appropriate).

Review Questions

1. What are minerals? Write down their importance.
2. How can we classify minerals based on their daily requirements?
3. What is the importance of calcium and its daily requirements for adults?
4. Write down the various functions, daily requirements and main food sources of iron and potassium.
5. What is ascorbic acid? Why do we need to consume it on daily basis?

Vitamins

Introduction

Vitamins are the organic compounds that are necessary in small amounts in animal and human diets to sustain life and health. The "vita" part of the word "vitamin" means "life". They are vital and essential for life and health. Vitamins regulate metabolism, help in the growth and maintenance of the body and protect against diseases. They do not provide energy and are usually required as co-enzymes or precursors of co-enzymes.

Why are they called vitamins?

In 1912 Dr. Casimir Funk, a Polish biochemist, put forth the theory that foods contained essential chemical substances that were vital to life. He coined the term vitamines referring to them as "vital amines", or nitrogen compounds. In fact, his 1922 work was titled "The Vitamines". It later turned out that some of these substances were not amines and the "e" was dropped. The term vitamin has been part of our nomenclature ever since.

Classification

Vitamins are classified according to how they are absorbed and stored in the body. There are two types of vitamins:

a) **Fat-soluble vitamins** include vitamins A, D, E and K.

b) **Water-soluble vitamins** include vitamins B-complex, C.

The body can store fat-soluble vitamins in the liver and fatty tissues. So their deficiency is not effective for long times. But most of the water-soluble vitamins are excreted out in the urine, so these should be consumed more often.

Fat Soluble Vitamins

The four fat-soluble vitamins i.e. A, D, E and K dissolve in fat but not in water. They are stored in the liver. They play important roles in the growth and maintenance of the body. Their presence affects the health and function of the eyes, skin, gastro intestinal tract, lungs, bones, teeth, nervous system and blood. As the body stores these vitamins, toxicity is possible.

While taking them as supplements, they need to be taken with the meals containing fats and minerals to be properly dissolved and digested before they can be absorbed.

Vitamin A

Synonyms: Vitamin A group includes Retinol, Retinal and Retinoic Acid. Their parent substance is beta-Carotene, which is known as a provitamin. Also called anti infection vitamin, anti xerophthalmic vitamin. The chemical name retinol was given to vitamin A, because it has a major function in the retina of the eye. Vitamin A was the first fat-soluble vitamin to be discovered by Mc Collum.

Sources: It is available in two forms: preformed vitamin A, known as retinol, which is found only in foods of animal origin, and pro-vitamin A, which is obtained from fruits and vegetables, and also called beta-carotene.

Fish liver oils, cod liver oil, animal liver, egg yolk, milk, and milk products—especially margarine that is usually fortified, Vegetables and fruits such as carrots, tomatoes, papaya, mango etc. are good sources of vitamin A. The availability of beta-carotene from the food varies from 25 to 50 percent, depending on the fat content of the diet. One unit of beta-carotene in foods is assumed to yield only 0.25 units of retinol. The requirement of beta-carotene will be therefore 4 times the requirement of retinol.

As vitamin A is fat-soluble, it is lost when milk is skimmed. In vegetables, Vitamin A exists as a provitamin in the form of Beta-carotenes, which are yellow pigments in the fruits and vegetables.

Daily Requirements: About 2 mg.

Functions:

- It is necessary for rhodopsin of rod cells and iodopsin of cone cells of the retina of eye. Rhodopsin and iodopsin are retinal pigments. Thus vitamin A promotes normal vision.
- It is also required for the normal growth and development of lacrimal glands (tear glands).
- It is also essential for the maintenance of epithelial cells of skin and mucous membrane. Healthy epithelial cells do not allow infection, which is why vitamin A is also called anti-infection vitamin.
- It promotes growth of bones and teeth.
- It is necessary for reproduction.
- Vitamin A has anti-cancer property.
- Retinol in the lowest oxidation state, probably, serves as hormone.

Deficiency Symptoms (Effects of Deficiency)

i) Nyctalopia (Night blindness)

ii) Xerophthalamia—Drying of eyeball

iii) Dermatitis—Dry and scaly skin

iv) Keratomalacia—Corneal epithelium becomes keratinized and opaque and may become softened and ulcerated

Excess Intakes

Hypervitaminosis A—If vitamin A is taken in excess it causes headache, nausea (discomfort preceding vomiting), vomiting, drowsiness, loss of appetite and pain in bones. Excess vitamin A during pregnancy can cause birth defects. Vitamin A content in supplements needs to be checked and also the intake of liver should be restricted to once a fortnight. There is no need to restrict beta carotene (fruits and vegetables).

Destroyed by: Strong light.

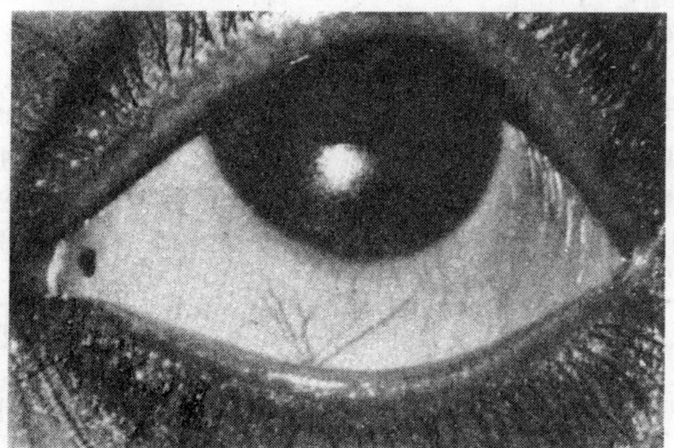

Xerophthalmia

Vitamin D

Synonyms: Anti rachitic vitamin, sunshine vitamin. Vitamin D exists in two forms:

Vitamin D2 (Ergocalciferol)—a synthetic derivative of a plant sterol.

Vitamin D3 (Cholecalciferol)—a derivative of cholesterol.

Sources: Egg yolk, milk, butter and fish liver oils contain vitamin D. The highest amount of vitamin D is present in fish liver oils (e.g., cod liver oil). Vitamin D is usually found in large quantities in the same foodstuffs, as vitamin A. Vitamin D is not actually a true vitamin because it is made in the body with the help of the sun's UV rays. The compound actually made in the skin is a prohormone. This irradiated compound in the skin has been given the name cholecalciferol, often shortened to calciferol because it is a fat soluble sterol that controls calcium metabolism in bone building. Vitamin D does not act directly in the body. It is first converted into 25 hydroxy cholecalciferol in the liver and subsequently to 1,25-dihydroxy cholecalciferol (DHCC) in the kidney. 1,25-DHCC is the active form of this vitamin, which functions in the body.

This vitamin is also formed in the skin by the UV rays present in sunlight, which converts a cholesterol derivative β-dehydrocholesterol present in the skin to vitamin D.

Daily Requirements

For better calcium absorption, 10 mg for infants and growing children is required. In tropical countries with plenty of sunlight, smaller amounts may suffice. Adults need less amounts of vitamin D.

Functions

1) Vitamin D promotes the absorption of calcium and phosphorous by the intestine.
2) It maintains the normal functioning of parathormone (hormone secreted by parathyroid glands).

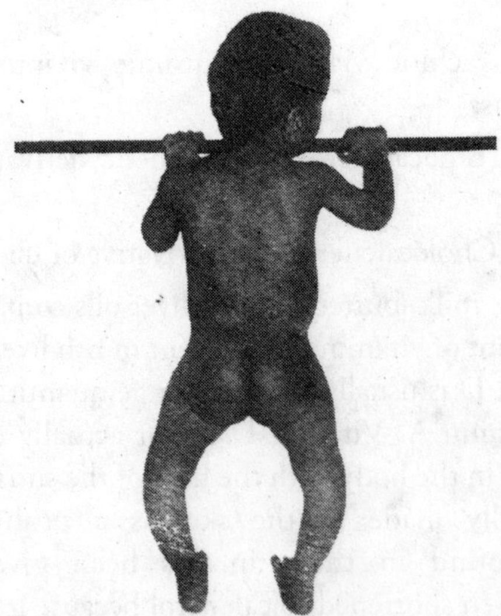

Rickets

3) It affects the metabolism of citric acid, which is a normal constituent of many body tissues including bones.

4) It exerts an anti-rachitic effect. Because it regulates metabolism of calcium and phosphorus, it affects normal growth of the body and formation of teeth and bones.

Deficiency Symptoms (Effects of Deficiency)

i. Rickets in children (softness and deformities of bones like bow-legs and pigeon-chest).

ii. Osteomalacia in adults (weak bones liable to easy fracture).

iii. Dental caries (cavities in teeth).

Excess Intakes: Hypervitaminosis D- if vitamin D is taken in excess it causes hypercalcemia (abnormally high blood calcium), hyper-phosphatemia (elevated blood phosphate levels), anorexia (loss of appetite), nausea, vomiting and diarrhoea. Too much vitamin D from supplements is dangerous.

Destroyed by: Oral contraceptives.

Vitamin E

Synonyms: Tocopherol, Anti-sterility vitamin, Fertility vitamin, vitamin of Reproduction, Beauty vitamin etc. Today, at least eight naturally occurring tocopherols are alpha, beta, gamma, zeta 1, zeta 2, eta, delta and epsilon. Alpha tocopherol has the highest vitamin activity.

Sources: Tocopherols are known to occur in a variety of plant and animal tissues. The most important natural sources of tocopherols are vegetable oils, of these wheat germ has the highest concentration. Soybeans, unrefined corn oils, cotton seed oil, safflower oil, broccoli, brussel sprouts, green leafy vegetables, sunflower seeds, sesame seeds, peanuts, whole grain cereals, tuna, sardines etc. are good sources of vitamin E. Liver is usually the highest in vitamin E content. Tocopherols are also found in animal body fat (adipose tissue).

Daily Requirements: About 15 to 20 mg.

Functions

- Tocopherols are excellent antioxidants and thus maintain normal bio membrane structure. It inhibits oxidation of unsaturated fatty acids and vitamin A.
- It keeps the skin healthy.
- It also decreases fragility (weakness) of the erythrocytes (RBCs). Thus its deficiency also causes anaemia in which RBCs are devoid of haemoglobin.
- Vitamin E has anti-cancer property. It is used for curing cancer.
- It maintains normal functioning of reproductive organs hence it is called Fertility vitamin.
- It maintains the muscles of the body, therefore, vitamin E should be a part of athlete's diet.
- It is also used to prevent heart attacks and treat Alzheimer's disease in some patients.
- It helps in the development and cell formation. Thus it is needed in the diet of pregnant, lactating women and for the newborn infants, particularly premature infants.
- It is required for proper use of vitamin A in the body.

Deficiency Symptoms (Effects of Deficiency)

1) Reproductive failure.
2) Degeneration of muscles (muscular dystrophy)—a degenerative disease of skeletal muscles.
3) Increased haemolysis (breakdown of erythrocytes-RBCs) leading to macrocytic anaemia (RBCs become larger).
4) Slow growth and degeneration of the renal tubules.
5) Easy bruising, exhaustion after light exercise, slow wound healing, lack of sex drive, varicose veins and loss of muscle tone.

Excess Intakes

Hypervitaminosis symptoms of vitamin E have not been reported yet. Extremely high doses of vitamin E may interfere with the blood-clotting action of vitamin K and enhance the effects of drugs used to oppose blood-clotting, causing haemorrhage.

Destroyed by: Heat

Vitamin K

Synonyms: Antihaemorrhagic factor, Antihaemorrhagic vitamin, Coagulation vitamin, Phylloquinone.

Sources: Alfalfa grass (a plant used for fodder), spinach, cauliflower, cabbage, tomato, soybeans, wheat bran, wheat germ, whole wheat, vegetable oils, liver, pork, fish etc. It is synthesized by bacteria in the large intestine (colon). Vitamin K is of two types: vitamin K1 and vitamin K2. The vitamin K1 is abundant in vegetable oils, leafy green vegetables and wheat bran, whereas, vitamin K2 is synthesized by the intestinal bacteria.

One cup of green tea, made from leaves, provides a good amount of vitamin K. As well as being an effective antioxidant, green tea is a healthy alternative to coffee or tea,

Daily Requirements: About 0.07 to 0.14 mg.

Functions

1) It is necessary for the synthesis of prothrombin, the precursor of thrombin, one of the factors needed for the normal coagulatory function of the blood. A blood clot is made up of fibrin, a protein, which is deposited as fine threads to form a network. The formation of fibrin from fibrinogen requires thrombin and the formation of thrombin from prothrombin requires calcium and vitamin K. Vitamin K is an essential part of the enzyme system involved in the production of the blood clotting factor. Thus vitamin K helps in blood clotting, prevention of haemorrhage and excessive bleeding of wounds.

Prothrombin + Calcium + Vitamin K = Thrombin
Thrombin + Fibrinogen = Fibrin (blood clot)

2) It helps in preventing internal bleeding, haemorrhages and aids in reducing excessive menstrual flow.
3) It also participates in the synthesis of bone proteins and may help protect against hip fractures.

Deficiency Symptoms (Effects of Deficiency)

Vitamin K deficiency causes a decrease in the prothrombin content of the blood, thus resulting in faulty blood clotting and a tendency to bleeding (haemorrhages) increases.

Excess Intakes

Hypervitaminosis K: Excess intake of vitamin K causes gastrointestinal disturbance and anaemia.

Destroyed by: Prolonged use of antibiotics and sulpha drugs.

Water Soluble Vitamins

Water-soluble vitamins are soluble in water. Because of their water solubility, water-soluble vitamins except vitamin B_{12} have no stable storage form and must be provided continuously in the diet. All water soluble vitamins except vitamin C act as coenzymes or cofactors in enzymatic reactions.

Vitamin B-complex

Vitamin B-complex is generally found in germinating seeds, wheat germ, pulses, beans and lentils, yeast, liver and meat. Bacteria of intestine mostly synthesize them. Vitamin B-complex includes the seven B vitamins namely Thiamine (B_1), riboflavin (B_2), niacin (B_3), pantothenic acid (B_5), pyridoxine (B_6), folic acid (B_9) and cobalamin (B_{12}), which are as follows :

Vitamin B_1

Synonyms: Thiamine, Anti-neuritic vitamin, Anti-beriberi substance, Aneurine.

Sources: Thiamine occurs in the outer coats of seeds of many plants including the cereal grains. Unpolished rice and food made of whole grains are good sources of this vitamin. It is also synthesized by bacteria in the colon.

Daily Requirements: About 1.2 to 1.5 mg

Functions:

i. Thiamine serves as a coenzyme in the chemical pathway responsible for the metabolism of carbohydrates. Thiamine deficiency interferes with the metabolism of glucose and the production of energy.

ii. It is essential for amino acid metabolism.

iii. It plays an important role in tissue respiration, tones the nervous system and muscles, improves appetite and promotes growth.

Deficiency Symptoms (Effects of Deficiency)

Deficiency of vitamin B_1 causes Beriberi. This disease mainly occurs among people subsisting on a polished rice diet. This disease is rare in the Western world because of food habits and food enrichment. Beriberi is a condition caused by severe prolonged deficiency of vitamin B_1, characterized by neurological symptoms, cardiovascular abnormalities, and oedema. Beriberi refers to a constellation of heart, gastrointestinal, and nervous system problems from thiamine deficiency.

Four major types of beriberi exist

1. **Wet beriberi**, which affects primarily the cardiovascular system;

Symptoms of wet beriberi include:

- Fast heart rate
- Swollen feet and legs
- Enlarged heart
- Enlarged, tender liver
- Shortness of breath
- Congestion in the lungs

2. **Dry beriberi**, which affects primarily the nervous system;

Symptoms of dry beriberi include:

- Numbness, tingling, burning pain in extremities
- Pain and cramping in the leg muscles
- Difficulty with speech
- Problems in walking
- Disturbed sense of balance

3. **Shoshin**, which is a rapidly evolving and frequently fatal form of cardiovascular beriberi. Symptoms of shoshin beriberi are the same as those of wet beriberi, but the only difference is that its onset is sudden, the progression is rapid, and the risk of death is very high.

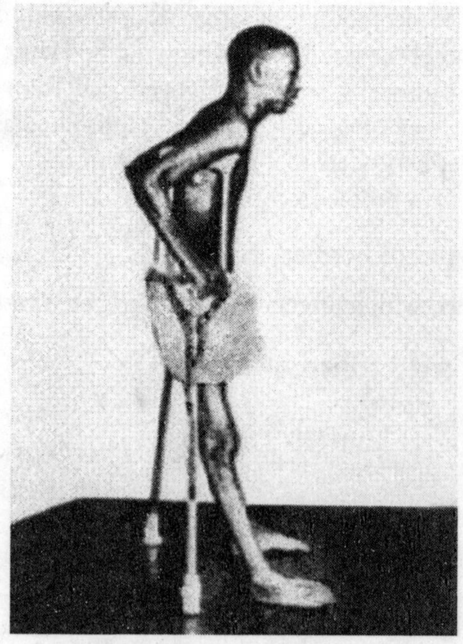

A typical case of Beri-Beri

4. **Infantile beriberi**, which tends to strike babies between the ages of one and four months who are breastfed by mothers who are severely thiamine deficient.

Symptoms of infantile beriberi include:

- Restlessness
- Difficulty in sleeping
- Diarrhea
- Swollen arms and legs
- Muscle wasting in arms and legs
- Silent cry
- Heart failure

The syndrome caused by thiamine deficiency in alcoholism is called **Wernicke-Korsakoff syndrome.**

Destroyed by: Cooking.

Vitamin B_2

Synonyms: Riboflavin, Lactoflavin (from milk), Ovaflavin (from egg yolk), Hepatoflavin (from liver) and Verdoflavin (from grass). Vitamin B2 is also called Vitamin G.

Sources: Riboflavin is synthesized by green plants, many bacteria (e.g., intestinal bacteria) and fungi but not by animals. Liver is a good source of this vitamin.

Daily Requirements: About 1.5 to 1.8 mg.

Functions

(i) This vitamin is essential for growth and health.

(ii) It maintains healthy skin and oral mucosa.

(iii) It is also associated with the physiology of vision.

(iv) Essential for converting carbohydrate into energy.

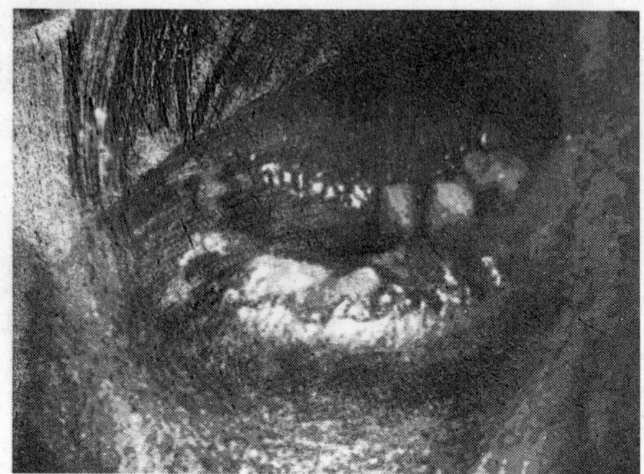

Cheilosis

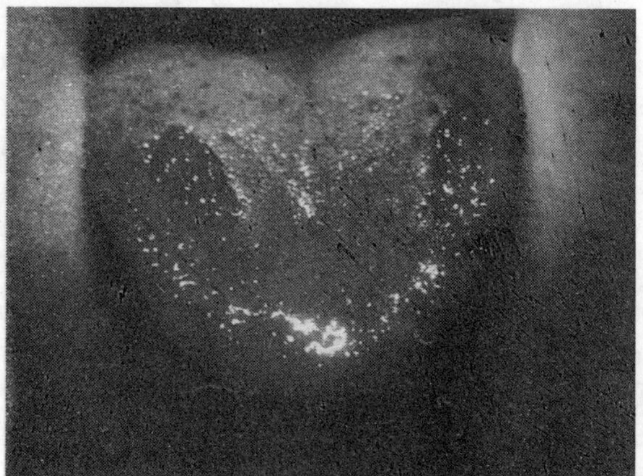

Glossitis

Source: Kathleen M.L., Page-106

Deficiency Symptoms (Effects of Deficiency)

Riboflavin deficiency results in poor growth and other pathological changes in the skin, eyes, liver, and nerves. Riboflavin deficiency in humans is usually associated with a cracking at the comers of the mouth called cheilosis, inflammation of the tongue, which appears red and glistening (glossitis), corneal vascularization accompanied by itching; and a scaly, greasy dermatitis about the corners of the nose, eyes, and ears. Other symptoms of the deficiency of riboflavin are digestive disorders, burning sensation in the skin and eyes, headache, mental depression, forgetfulness, scaly dermatitis at angles of nostrils and keratitis of cornea.

Destroyed by: Light.

Vitamin B_3

Synonyms: Niacin, Nicotinic acid, Nicotinamide, Pellagra preventing factor, Antipellagra factor.

Sources: This vitamin is found in plant and animal tissues. Animal organs like liver, kidney and some fish are outstanding sources of this vitamin. It is also synthesized by colon bacteria. Niacin can be formed in the body from the amino acid tryptophan, which is present in all dietary proteins. Sixty mg of this amino acid can give rise to 1 mg of nicotinic acid in the body.

Daily Requirements: About 15 to 20 mg.

Functions

1) This vitamin is necessary for the metabolism of carbohydrates.
2) It is also essential for the normal functioning of the gastrointestinal tract and the satisfactory functioning of the nervous system.

Deficiency Symptoms (Effects of Deficiency)

Its deficiency causes a disease called Pellagra (it is made up of an Italian word pelle which means skin and agra meaning rough, Pellagra = rough skin). It is characterized by three D's namely: Dermatitis (inflammation of skin which becomes scaly and papillated), Diarrohea (watery stool), and Dementia (mental deterioration which may lead to madness). Muscle atrophy and severe inflammation of mucous membrane of alimentary canal may occur.

Pellagra is especially frequent among people eating food with low tryptophan (an essential amino acid) content. Hartnup's disease, a

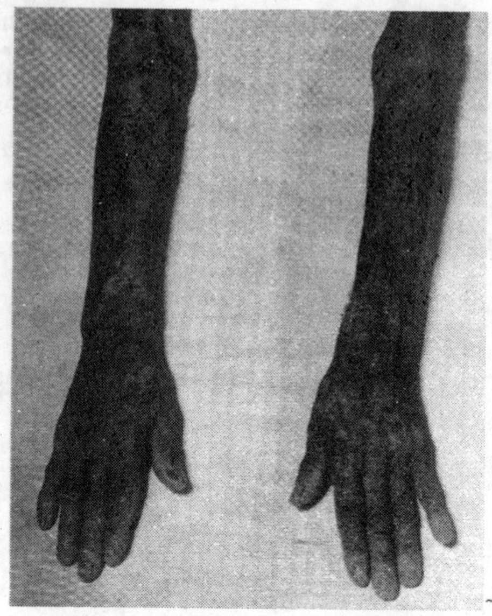

Pellagra

Source: Kathleen M.L., Page-101

hereditary abnormality in metabolism of tryptophan is characterized by pellagra like skin rash, temporary ataxia (loss of the power of muscular coordination) and mental deterioration. The urine of the patient of this disease contains increased amount of tryptophan.

Destroyed by: Cooking

Vitamin B_5

Synonyms: Pantothenic Acid

Sources: The word *Pantothenic* in Greek language means" from everywhere". Hence, it is widely distributed and is found in various foods. It is found in yeast, milk, ground nut, tomatoes, liver, meat, kidneys, egg etc. Its richest source is wheat germ and honey. Tea also contains fair amounts of this vitamin. It is also synthesized by bacteria in the colon.

Daily Requirements: 5 to 15 mg.

Functions:

1) This vitamin is essential for the healthy skin and hair.

2) It is required for the normal functioning of the adrenal glands.

Deficiency Symptoms (Effects of Deficiency)

As it is found in almost all food stuffs, its deficiency is rare in humans.

Destroyed by: Not established.

Vitamin B_6

Synonyms: Pyridoxine, Pyridoxal , Pyridoxamine, Adermin.

Sources: Egg yolk, milk, peas, beans, whole grain cereals, soybeans, yeast, green leafy vegetables, meat and liver. Intestinal bacteria also synthesize it.

Daily Requirements: About 2 mg.

Functions:

(i) The vitamin B_6 helps in the metabolism of amino acids.

(ii) Vitamin B_6 is useful in the treatment of nausea and vomiting during pregnancy (morning sickness), radiation sickness and muscular dystrophy.

(iii) It also maintains nervous system.

Deficiency Symptoms (Effects of Deficiency)

Pyridoxine is usually sufficient in the daily diet and it is also synthesized by the intestinal bacteria so human beings usually do not suffer from its deficiency. However, a widely used anti tuberculosis drug isoniazid induces a vitamin B_6 deficiency. The deficiency causes dermatitis, anaemia, convulsions, nausea, vomiting, mental disorders and retarded growth.

Destroyed by: Cooking and oral contraceptives.

Pyridoxine helps in the generation of **niacin** (nicotinic acid) from **tryptophan** and thus pyridoxine deficiency also causes pellagra.

Folic Acid

Synonyms: Folacin, folate, Vitamin M, Vitamin 10, Pteroyglutamic acid (PGA).

Sources: The major sources of folic acid are green leafy vegetables and other sources include liver, kidney, yeast and soybean etc. Folic acid is also synthesized by intestinal bacteria.

Daily Requirements: About 0.4 mg.

Functions

1. It helps in DNA synthesis,
2. It is also important for the growth and formation of RBCs.

Deficiency Symptoms (Effects of Deficiency)

Its deficiency causes macrocytic anaemia or megalobastic anaemia. Its deficiency also causes sprue (ulceration of mouth, inflammation of bowel (intestine), inability to absorb, especially fats and diarrhoea).

Destroyed by: Cooking

Vitamin B_{12}

Water-soluble vitamins except vitamin B_{12} have no stable storage form and must be provided continuously in the diet. Vitamin B_{12} can be stored in the liver.

Synonyms: Cyanocobalamin, Cobalamin, Anti-pernicious anaemia factor, Castle's intrinsic factor, Animal protein factor (APF).

Sources: Vitamin B_{12} is a dark red compound containing cobalt. It is not found in plants. However, it is considered that Spirulina (an alga) contains vitamin B_{12}. Strict vegetarians may be at risk of vitamin B_{12} deficiency. Liver and kidneys are the richest sources and milk, meat, fish and eggs are good sources of this vitamin. It is also synthesized by intestinal bacteria, which infact, are main sources of vitamin B_{12}.

Daily Requirements: 3μg

Functions

(i) Vitamin B_{12} plays an important role in the synthesis of nucleic acid (e.g. DNA).

(ii) It stimulates the bone marrow to produce RBCs. Thus it is important for the formation and maturation of RBCs.

Deficiency Symptoms (Effects of Deficiency)

Deficiency of vitamin B_{12} leads to pernicious (injurious) anaemia (greater decrease in the number of RBCs formation in the bone marrow). Pernicious anemia refers to a type of autoimmune anaemia which causes a fall in the number of red blood cells. The formation of the red blood cells depends on the adequate absorption of vitamin B_{12}, which depends upon the presence of the 'intrinsic factor', which is secreted by the stomach lining. If the secretion of this substance stops, it will never restart and the treatment of this condition is injections of vitamin B_{12}, which will be required for the patients' remaining life span. Its deficiency disturbs normal synthesis of nucleic acids particularly DNA. Its deficiency also causes nervous disorders.
Destroyed by: Excessive heat.

Choline

Choline is important for the structural integrity of the cell membranes, the breakdown and utilization of fat for energy, cholesterol transport and elimination from the body. Choline is significant for communicating information from nerve to nerve and also plays an important role in male and female fertility. It is very important for proper cognitive development in newborns.

Sources: The best sources are lecithin granules, desiccated liver, eggs, fish, liver, wheat germ and brewer's yeast.

Deficiency Symptoms (Effects of Deficiency)

No specific symptoms, but lack of this vitamin can lead to fatty liver, nerve degeneration, high blood pressure, atherosclerosis, thrombosis, high blood cholesterol, senile dementia and reduced resistance to infection.

Inositol

Inositol and choline work together closely to make neurotransmitters and the fatty substances in the cell membranes, they also combine to move fats out of life. It is present in muscles and liver. Its absence from the diet causes alopecia (loss of hair).

Sources: Most people get about 1,000 mg a day from their food. Phytic acid, a substance found in the fibre of plants, gets turned into inositol when bacteria in the intestine digest it. Other good sources include organ meats, citrus fruits, nuts, beans and whole grains.

Deficiency Symptoms (Effects of Deficiency): Deficiency is unlikely.

PABA–Para–Amino Benzoic Acid

PABA is not a B vitamin but it does make part of the folic acid molecule and can therefore be classed as an unofficial B vitamin. It blocks ultra-violet radiations from sunlight that is why it is an ingredient in sunscreens and shampoos. It helps restores hair to its natural color and relieves arthritis.

Sources: Liver, wheat germ, brown rice and whole grains.

Deficiency Symptoms (Effects of Deficiency): It is not usually seen.

Biotin

Synonyms: Vitamin H, Vitamin B_7, Anti-egg white injury factor, Coenzyme R.

Sources: Yeast, liver, egg yolk, tomatoes, honey. It is also supplied from the intestinal bacteria.

Daily Requirements: 150 to 300 μg

Functions

1) It serves as coenzyme needed for protein and fatty acid synthesis.
2) Helps in maintaining healthy skin, hair, sweat glands, nerves and bone marrow.

Deficiency Symptoms (Effects of Deficiency)

Its deficiency does not occur normally because a large portion of the human biotin requirement is supplied from the intestinal bacteria. However, prolonged use of anti-bacterial drugs (e.g., antibiotics and sulpha drugs) reduce the intestinal flora and may cause its deficiency. Biotin deficiency causes skin lesions, poor growth, loss of muscular control, loss of appetite, weakness, hair fall etc.

> Biotin deficiency also occurs by eating raw egg white in large quantities, as the raw egg white contains avidin protein which prevents the absorption of biotin. Therefore, egg should never be eaten raw.

Destroyed by: The intake of raw egg white which contains avidin prevents absorption of biotin. It can be easily prevented by boiling the egg before feeding.

Vitamin C

Synonyms: Ascorbic acid, antiscorbic vitamin.

Sources: Citrus fruits (e.g., lemon and orange), amla, guava, tomato, potato, peppers, fresh green vegetables and salad vegetables like cabbage, lettuce, sprouted beans and pulses, spinach, etc. Amla is the richest source of natural vitamin C.

Daily Requirements: 50 mg

> Vitamin C was the earliest known vitamin. It is the most sensitive of all vitamins to heat and was the first vitamin to be produced during fermentation process using Acetobacter, a wild bacterium by Albert Gyorgi.

Functions

(i) Vitamin C helps in the formation of collagen, bone matrix, tooth dentine and other extra cellular materials.

(ii) It is necessary for healthy gums and teeth.

(iii) It helps in the proper absorption and utilization of iron in the body.

(iv) It helps in the production of antibodies and for the formation of RBCs.

(v) It helps in healing wounds and helps body to withstand injury from burns and toxicity.

(vi) It has antioxidant property.

(vii) It helps in the metabolism of many acids.

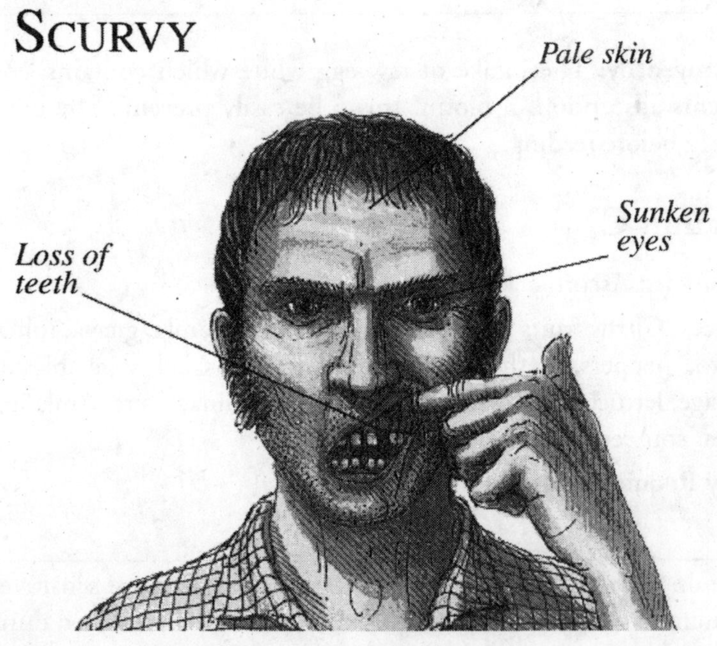

Deficiency Symptoms (Effects of deficiency)

Vitamin C deficiency causes scurvy which is characterized by spongy and bleeding gums, loose and falling teeth, fragility of blood capillaries, fragile bones, delay in wound healing, swollen and painful joints, mild anaemia and nervous disorder. People depending solely upon milk, meat, eggs and cereals usually suffer from scurvy. Vegetable eaters never get scurvy.

Excess Intakes

When excess of vitamin C is taken some amount of ascorbic acid is converted into oxalic acid, which can cause stone formation in the kidney and urinary tract.

Destroyed by: Heat and light.

Vitamin P

Synonyms: Hesperidin, Citrin, Rutin.

Sources: Citrus fruits, green vegetables, lemon rind and rinds of fruits and vegetables are good sources of hesperidin. Buckwheat (wild wheat) leaves are good source of rutin.

Functions: It helps in maintaining resistance in the walls of blood capillaries.

Review Questions

1. What are vitamins? Discuss water and fat-soluble vitamins.
2. Write down various fat-soluble vitamins and their functions.
3. Enlist various B-complex vitamins and their daily requirements.
4. What are non-official vitamins?
5. Write down various vitamins and their deficiency diseases?

6 Nutrient-Drug Interactions and Food

Introduction

Medicine serves to help people when they are sick, allowing them to live longer and healthier lives. Medications have become an integral part of life for many people. With rapidly growing research and technology, medications are more beneficial, and new ones continue to be discovered. Drugs do need to be taken with caution. All medications, whether prescribed by a doctor or bought over-the-counter, are capable of harmful side effects. The foods people eat contain nutrients that are used by the body to produce energy. Sometimes, certain medications may interact with both the food eaten and the nutrients the food gives to the body for proper functioning. A nutrient-drug interaction occurs, when the body is unable to use a nutrient due to a drug.

Generic Drugs

Generic drugs often are substituted for brand-name counterparts. They usually are more economical than brand-name drugs. Possible exceptions might be enteric-coated aspirin.

Patients may have concerns about the quality, efficacy, potency or consistency of generic drugs. Generics are therapeutically equivalent to brands approved and rated by the Food and Drug Administration. Major brand-name companies make many of these.

Over-the-Counter Drugs

- OTC drugs usually are meant only to relieve symptoms, not cure a disease or illness.
- Improper use can make symptoms worse or conceal a serious condition that should be brought to a doctor's attention. Never take OTC drugs longer than recommended on the label. If symptoms persist or if new symptoms occur, one should always see a doctor.
- Read the label carefully before taking an OTC product. There may be important changes in indications, warnings or directions.
- People with allergies or chronic health problems should be especially careful to read the ingredient, warning and caution statements carefully.
- Check expiration dates from time to time. Destroy in the safest way, any drugs that are outdated or that have deteriorated, such as discolored eye drops or ointment etc.
- When pregnant or nursing a baby, check with a health professional before taking any drugs.
- Drugs are either analgesic (pain control) or antipyretic (fever control).

Functions of a Drug

A drug is taken to prevent or treat sickness and disease. It is important to know what happens in the body when a drug is taken in order to better understand the interaction between nutrients and drugs. The action of a drug taken orally generally occurs in four steps: (1) the drug dissolves in the stomach, (2) the drug is absorbed into the blood and moves via the blood to the area of the body that needs it, (3) the body reacts to the medicine, and (4) the body gets rid of the drug by way of the kidney, liver, or both.

Nutrient-Drug Interactions

Drug	Indication	Possible Effects Type of
Coumadin	Anticoagulant (blood thinner)	Vitamin K is a nutrient in the body that helps blood to clot. Vitamin K is present in foods such as green leafy vegetables and fish. It interferes with a blood thinner like coumadin.
Dilantin	Anticonvulsant (anti-seizure)	Vitamin D and folic acid levels in the body are decreased by the consumption of these types of drugs.
Norvasc	Antihypertensive (for high blood pressure)	Consuming foods high in sodium decrease the effectiveness of the drug.
Aspirin	Anti-inflammatory/ pain reliever	Taking large amounts of these drugs will cause a loss of Vitamin C in the body
Birth control pills	Oral contraceptives	Women who take these drugs often have low levels of folic acid and Vitamin B_6 in the blood.
Dyazide/ Thiazide	Diuretics (water-eliminating)	Taking diuretics often leads to a loss of potassium in the body.
Tetracycline	Antibiotic	Calcium may interact with the effectiveness of the antibiotic. Avoid dairy products for two to three hours before and after taking the medicine.
Lipitor/ Zocor	Statins (cholesterol-lowering drugs)	Antioxidants (Vitamin A, C, E, B, folic acid) may interact with the drug by reversing its effect.
Prednisone	Corticosteroid	The drug may increase appetite thus increasing nutrient intake.

Adverse effects of Nutrient-Drug Interactions

A nutrient-drug interaction may influence the body in several ways. Certain foods can affect the rate at which the body uses a medication. A drug will not work as well if a certain nutrient in a food speeds up or slows down drug's absorption into the body. Short or long-term instances of nutrient-drug interactions may be life threatening. A nutrient-drug interaction may also impact the nutritional status of the body. Nutrient-drug interactions can occur with both prescription and over-the-counter medicine.

Impact of Food on Effectiveness of a Drug

A medication has ingredients, just as food does, that allow it to function correctly when taken in order to help the body in some way. A food may interfere with the effectiveness of a drug if the food interacts with the ingredients in the medication, preventing the drug from working properly. Nutrients in food may either delay absorption into the body or speed up elimination from the body, either or which can impact a drug's effectiveness. For example, the acidic ingredients in fruit juices are capable of decreasing the power of antibiotics such as penicillin. Tetracycline, another infection-fighting drug, is impacted by the consumption of dairy products. Many medications that are taken to fight depression can be dangerous if mixed with beverages or foods that consist of tyramine, which is found in items such as beer, red wine, and some cheeses.

Food can also impact the effectiveness of a drug due to the way it is consumed. Generally, medicine is to be taken at the same time food is eaten. This is because the medicine may upset the stomach if the stomach is empty. However, sometimes taking a drug at the same time that food is eaten can interfere with the way the medicine is absorbed by the body.

Impact on Nutritional Status

A drug has the capacity of interfering with a person's nutritional status. Appetite may be stimulated by a certain drug, resulting in an increase in nutrient intake due to more food being eaten. However, drugs may also decrease appetite, leading to a decrease in nutrient intake. In this case, a drug could possibly cause a nutritional deficiency. Nutritional status may also be impacted by a drug's effect on the three main nutrients: carbohydrates, fat, and protein. A drug may speed up or slow down the breakdown of these three nutrients, which are essential to the body's functioning. When a drug affects the absorption of nutrients from food into the body, less energy is available to be used by the body. The impact of the nutrient-drug interaction may vary according to the medicine taken, the dose of the medicine given, and the form taken (e.g., pill, liquid).

The Elderly and Nutrient-Drug Interactions

Elderly persons are at a significant risk for nutrient-drug interactions. This population often takes the highest amount of medications, and with the use of multiple drugs, certain problems may exist. A loss of appetite, a reduced sense of taste and smell, and swallowing problems all may result from medication which are given to elderly people.

Malnutrition is a common problem among older adults. Therefore, nutritional status may be already impacted by decreased nutrient intake. This may only worsen the effect of a possible nutrient-drug interaction. Elderly people who take many drugs on a routine basis for long periods of time are at greatest risk of nutrient depletion and nutritional deficiencies.

Avoid Nutrient-Drug Interactions

There are ways to avoid placing the body at risk of an unwanted nutrient-drug interaction. The following are tips to remember about taking medications and will help avoid interactions:

- Be sure to read the label on a prescription medicine and ask a pharmacist or physician if something is not clear.
- Read all directions, warnings, and any possible side effects printed on all drug labels and information in the package.

- Always take medications with a full glass of water.
- A drug may not work correctly if a medicine is taken improperly; do not stir medication into food or take apart capsules (unless told to do so).
- Take vitamin and mineral supplements before or after medicine, as they may interact with certain drugs.
- Avoid stirring drugs into hot drinks such as coffee because the drug's effectiveness can be destroyed by the hot temperature.
- Do not drink alcohol when taking any medicine.
- Always tell a physician and pharmacist about all medicines being taken, including both prescription and over-the-counter drugs.
- Medications need to be taken at different times relative to meals.

Review Questions

1. What are generic and over the counter drugs?
2. Explain nutrient drug interactions.
3. What impact do the drugs have on our life?
4. Does our nutritional status get affected by the drugs?
5. What points should be kept in mind to avoid nutrient drug interactions?

		Use	Interactions/ Guidelines
ALLERGIES	Antihistamine	To relieve or prevent the symptoms of colds, hay fever and allergies.	**FOOD**: Take prescription on an empty stomach to increase its effectiveness. ALCOHOL: Avoid alcohol because it increases the sedative effects of the medications.
ARTHRITIS and PAIN	Analgesic/ Antipyretic	To treat mild to moderate pain and fever	**FOOD:** For rapid relief, take on empty stomach. ALCOHOL: Avoid or limit the use of alcohol because chronic alcohol use can increase the risk of liver damage or stomach bleeding.
	Corticosteroids	To relieve inflamed areas of the body. To reduce swelling and itching. To help relieve allergies, rheumatoid arthritis, and other conditions	**FOOD:** Take with food or milk to decrease stomach upset.
	Narcotic Analgesic	To provide relief for moderate to severe pain.	**ALCOHOL:** Avoid alcohol because it increases the sedative effects of the medication.
ASTHMA	Bronchodilators	To treat the symptoms of bronchial asthma, chronic bronchitis and emphysema.	**FOOD:** High-fat meals may increase the amount of theophylline in the body, while high-carbohydrate meals may decrease it **CAFFEINE:** Avoid eating or drinking large amounts of foods and beverages that contain caffeine. **ALCOHOL:** Avoid alcohol because it can

		Use	Interactions/ Guidelines
			increase the risk of side effects such as nausea, vomiting, headache and irritability
CARDIO-VASCULAR DISORDERS	Diuretics	To help eliminate water, sodium and chloride from the body.	**FOOD:** Some diuretics cause loss of potassium, calcium and magnesium. Triamterene is known as a "potassium sparing" diuretic. When taking triamterene avoid eating large amounts of potassium-rich foods such as bananas, oranges and green leafy vegetables or salt substitutes.
	Beta Blockers	To decrease the nerve impulses to blood vessels.	**ALCOHOL:** Avoid drinking alcohol with propranolol/inderal because these drugs lower blood pressure too much.
	Nitrates	To relax blood vessels and lower the demand for oxygen by the heart	**ALCOHOL**: Avoid alcohol because it may add to the blood vessel-relaxing effect of nitrates and result in dangerously low blood pressure.
	Anticoagulants	To prevent the formation of blood clots.	**FOOD:** Vitamin K produces blood-clotting substances and may reduce the effectiveness of anticoagulants. High doses of vitamin E (400 IU or more) may prolong clotting time and increase the risk of bleeding.
INFECTIONS	Antibiotics and Antifungals	To treat infections caused by bacteria and fungi.	**GENERAL GUIDELINES:** Tell the doctor if Antifungals by bacteria and fungi. You experience skin rashes or diarrhea. If you are using birth control,

		Use	Interactions/ Guidelines
			consult with your health care provider because some methods may not work when taken with antibiotics. Be sure to finish all of your medication even if you start feeling better. Take medication with plenty of water.
	Antibacterials/ Penicillin	To treat infections caused by bacteria and fungi.	**FOOD:** Take on an empty stomach unless it upsets your stomach, then take with food.
	Tetracyclines	To treat infections caused by bacteria and fungi.	**FOOD:** Avoid taking tetracycline with dairy products, antacids, and vitamin supplements containing iron because they can interfere with the medication's effectiveness.
	Antifungals		**FOOD:** It is important to avoid taking these medications with dairy products. **ALCOHOL:** Avoid drinking alcohol and taking medications that contain alcohol while taking kerocon-zole and for at least three days after you finish the medication.
STOMACH CONDITIONS	Histamine Blockers	To relieve pain, promote healing and prevent irritation from returning.	**FOOD:** These mediations can be taken with or without food. **CAFFEINE:** Caffeine products may irritate the stomach.

Therapeutic Nutrition or Nutrition Therapy

Introduction

Therapeutic nutrition deals with the adequacy and modifications of diets during diseased conditions. Food plays an important and significant role in illness. Therapeutic diets are planned to maintain or restore good nutrition in the patients and used to supplement the medical treatment of the patient.

Objectives of Nutrition/Diet Therapy

There are various objectives of diet therapy which are as follows:

- Prevent/correct malnutrition and maintain good nutritional status.
- Prevent wasting of muscle, bone, blood, organs and other lean body mass.
- Help the patient tolerate treatment.
- Reduce nutrition-related side effects and complications.
- Maintain strength and energy.
- Increase immunity to fight against infections.
- Help recovery and healing.
- Maintain or improve quality of life.
- To correct nutrient deficiencies which occurred due to the disease.

- To afford rest to the whole body or to a particular organ affected by the disease.
- To bring about changes in the body weight whenever necessary.
- Intake of the food must be adjusted by the body to metabolize the nutrients during the disease.

Factors to be considered while Planning Therapeutic Diets

- The diseased condition, which need a change in the diet.
- Duration of the disease.
- The patient's tolerance for food.
- Economic status, liking and disliking of the patient should be considered.

Therapeutic Modifications of the Normal Diet

Therapeutic modifications are made according to disease, symptoms, condition of the patient and the metabolic changes. Commonly made therapeutic modifications are:

1. Consistency of the diet is changed as per the condition of the patient. The main motive is to provide changes in consistency, as in fluid and soft diets. There are many diseases like mouth ulcers, in which the patient cannot take solid foods and to such patients liquid or soft diets are suggested. Whereas, in other diseases like diabetes food of normal consistency is recommended.
2. Energy intakes are modified according to the physical state and disease of the patient. Energy intakes are usually decreased when the patient is at bed rest since long time or when the patient is obese or overweight. Depending upon the disease high or low energy diets are given.
3. In certain diseases, which are caused by the deficiency or excess of any specific nutrient, modifications in the content are made. Few

examples of these diets are low fat diet, low sodium diet, high carbohydrate diet etc.

4. For the patients who are unable to consume food orally, intravenous method or tube feeding is employed.
5. Sometimes therapeutic modifications also include inclusion or exclusion of certain food, frequency of feeding is adjusted and most often bland diets are given.

Mode of Feeding

The method of feeding used in the nutritional care plan depends on the patient's condition. The dietician and nurse work together to manage the diet by using enteral or parenteral feeding. Patient may be fed using enteral nutrition (through a tube inserted into the stomach or intestine) or parenteral nutrition (infused into the bloodstream directly). The nutrients are delivered in formulas, liquids that contain water, protein, fats, carbohydrates, vitamins and/or minerals. The content of the formula depends on the needs of the patient and the method of feeding.

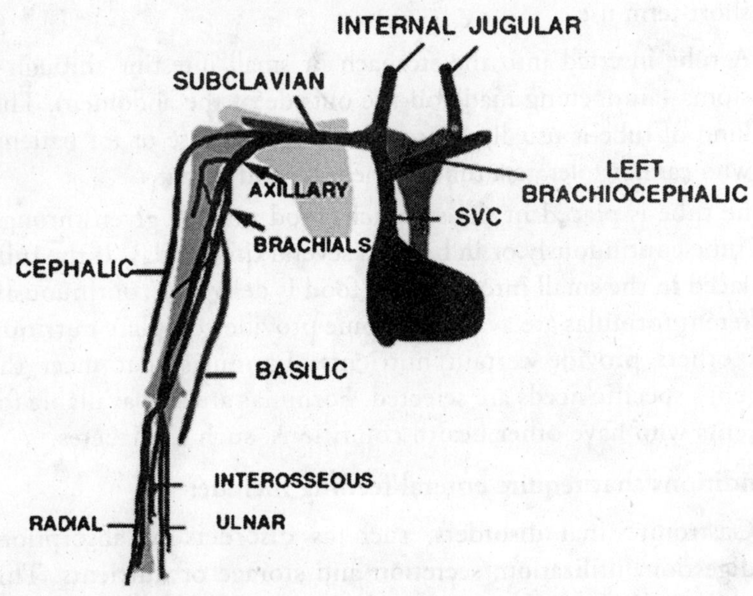

Enteral or Oral Feeding

Usually the regular oral feedings are the preferred methods of feeding as long as it is possible. If needed nutrient supplements can be added. The patient should always be encouraged to ingest food through the oral route.

Enteral (Tube) Feeding

Enteral feeding, or tube feeding, is used for the patients who have a functioning gastrointestinal tract, but are unable to orally ingest adequate nutrients to meet their metabolic needs. Enteral nutrition is food (in liquid form) given to the patient through a tube that is inserted into the stomach or the small intestine. The enteral feeding by the tube provides nutritional support. In this method of feeding a small tube is placed through the nasal cavity running down to the back of the throat into either the stomach or small intestine. Full fluid diets or commercial formulas may be administered through this route. The following types of tube feeding may be used:

- A tube inserted through the nose and throat down into the stomach or small intestine. This kind of tube is usually used for short-term use.
- A tube inserted into the stomach or small intestine through a stoma (an opening made on the outside of the abdomen). This kind of tube is usually chosen for long-term use or for patients who cannot tolerate a tube in the nose and throat.

If the tube is placed in the stomach, food may be given through the tube continuously or in batches several times a day. If the tube is placed in the small intestine, the food is delivered continuously. Different formulas are available. Some provide complete nutrition and others provide certain nutrients. Formulas that meet the patient's specific needs are selected. Formulas are also available for patients who have other health conditions, such as diabetes.

Conditions that require enteral feeding include:

1. Gastrointestinal disorders, such as disorders of absorption, digestion, utilization, secretion and storage of nutrients. This

includes anatomic disruptions such as tracheoesophageal fistula.

2. Cardiopulmonary disorders and other conditions of hypermetabolism such as burns and cancer.
3. Neuromuscular disorders, spinal cord defects, and cerebral palsy or damage to the central nervous system.
4. Failure to thrive.
5. Prematurity.

Enteral nutrition is not appropriate for the following patients:

- Patients whose stomach and intestines are not working or have been removed.
- Patients who have a blockage in the bowel.
- Patients who have severe nausea, vomiting, and/or diarrhea.
- Patients whose platelet count is low. Platelets are blood cells that help prevent bleeding by causing blood clots to form.
- Patients who have low levels of all blood cells (white blood cells, red blood cells, and platelets).

Advantages of enteral feeding

- Adequate nutrition can be easily given to the patient.
- Foods and drugs, which may not be liked by the patient, can be administered.
- Large quantity can be given daily.
- Comparatively economical.
- Give rise to fewer complications.
- Better tolerated and physiologically safer.

Disadvantages of Enteral Feeding

There are few disadvantages of enteral feeding. If the patient has gastroesophageal reflux, aggressive enteral feeding may increase the risk of vomiting. Other physical disadvantages are diarrhea, skin breakdown or anatomic disruption. Mechanical disadvantages include a dislodged or occluded feeding tube. Metabolic risks include hyperglycemia and hyperphosphatemia.

Parenteral Feeding or Vein Feeding

Parenteral nutrition is used when the patient cannot take food by mouth or by enteral feeding. Parenteral feeding bypasses the normal digestive system. Nutrients are delivered to the patient directly into the blood, through a catheter (thin tube) inserted into a vein. This mode of feeding is done through the peripheral veins. Patients with the following problems are given parenteral nutrition:

- Stomach and intestines that are not working or have been removed.
- Severe nausea, diarrhea, or vomiting.
- Severe sores in the mouth or esophagus.
- A fistula (hole) in the stomach or esophagus.
- Loss of body weight and muscle with enteral nutrition.

The catheter may be placed into a vein in the chest or in the arm.

A central venous catheter is placed beneath the skin and into a large vein in the upper chest. Placement of a central venous catheter is done by a surgeon.

A peripheral venous catheter is placed into a vein in the arm. Placement of a peripheral venous catheter is done by trained medical staff. This site may be used for short-term parenteral feeding.

The patient is checked often for infection or bleeding at the site (place) where the catheter enters the body.

There are two types of parenteral feeding:

Peripheral Vein Feeding

The nutrient and energy intake is limited in this mode of feeding. Various solutions of dextrose, amino acids, vitamins, minerals, lipids can be fed directly into the peripheral veins. A major surgery, traumatic injury may cause malnutrition in view of the increased demands. This mode of feeding is only used when the need for the nutrient support is not extensive or long term.

Central Vein Feeding or Total Parenteral Nutrition (TPN)

If the intravenous therapy is to be carried out for longer time, then peripheral veins are unsuitable. So a larger central vein is selected in which with the help of a surgical procedure, a catheter is inserted into the subclavian vein for easy access. The use of the large central vein to deliver life-sustaining nourishment avoids the complications of vascular inflammation and thrombosis.

A team of specialists work together to administer the parenteral nutrition. Throughout this process patient needs special care and support. This mode of parenteral feeding allows for higher volumes of nutrients and can be used for long time. TPN provides all nutrients in a concentrated form to avoid fluid overload.

Diets used in the Hospitals

While making therapeutic modifications mostly the consistency of the diet is changed. The consistency of the diet is modified usually depending upon the physical state of the patient. These diets include regular, general or full diet. According to the patient's tolerance, diets are modified to soft, liquid, or semi solid diet.

Fluid Diets

When the patient is unable to tolerate solid food, fluid diets are given e.g. in febrile disorders, after operations etc. These diets are free from mechanical or chemical irritants. The degree of nutritional adequacy of these diets depends upon the type of fluid permitted. There are two types of fluid diets:

- Clear fluid diets
- Full fluid diet

Clear Fluid Diet

This type of diet consists of clear fluids. It is used whenever, an acute illness or surgery produces intolerance for food as shown by nausea, vomiting, anorexia and diarrhoea. In acute inflammatory conditions of the intestinal tract, following operations upon the colon or rectum when it is desirable to prevent evacuation from the bowel, clear fluid diet is suggested. In this condition nutrients have to be restricted. The diet given to the patient should be non-gas forming, non-irritating and non-stimulating to peristaltic action. In such conditions of the patient, clear fluid diets are helpful in preventing dehydration and maintaining water and electrolyte balance. This diet is nutritionally inadequate as it is deficient in proteins, minerals, vitamins and calories. So it is used for very short period of time. It should not be continued for more than 24 to 48 hours. It contains 300 to 500 kcal, 2 to 5 g proteins and negligible fat. This diet is usually given in 1 to 2 hour intervals.

Foods Allowed

Cereal and pulse waters, carbonated beverages, weak tea or coffee without milk, broths, strained juices etc. Fats are avoided.

Full Fluid Diets

These full fluid diets include all liquid foods. Full fluid diet bridges the gap between clear fluid diet and soft diet. This diet is recommended for the patients who are acutely ill and are unable to chew or swallow solid foods. This diet does not contain irritating fibre, condiments and spices. It is given to the patient after operations, in acute gastritis, acute infections and in diarrhoea. This diet is nutritionally adequate. Full fluid diet can be used for long periods in comparison to the clear fluid diets. Vitamin and mineral supplements can be added to the fluids to enhance the nutritive value. The average nutritional composition of this diet is approximately 1200 to 1800 Kcal, 35 to 60 gm of protein with adequate minerals and vitamins.

Foods Allowed

Strained vegetables and fruit juices, clear broths, strained cream soups, strained cereal and pulse gruels, milk and milk beverages, carbonated beverages, sugar, butter, cream, oil, cocoa and salt.

Regular Normal Diet

A normal diet is one, which is made up of all foods eaten by the person in health. It is most frequently used in all the hospitals. It is used for bed patients who do not need a special diet. Many special diets progress ultimately to a regular diet.

Soft Diet

The soft diet serves as a transition from liquids to a regular diet for individuals who are recovering from surgery or a long illness. It can help to ease difficulty in chewing or swallowing due to dental problems or extreme weakness, and it is sometimes recommended to relieve mild intestinal or stomach discomfort. The soft diet can be especially helpful to patients who are undergoing treatments like chemotherapy, or radiation to the head, neck or abdominal areas, which may cause digestive problems or make the mouth and throat sore.

The soft diet limits or eliminates foods that are hard to chew and swallow, such as raw fruits and vegetables, meats etc. In some cases, high-fiber foods like whole-grain breads and cereals and "gas-forming" vegetables like broccoli or cauliflower are restricted to facilitate digestion. Fried and highly seasoned or spicy foods may also be limited. Foods are usually softened by cooking or mashing.

This diet gives 1500 to 2000 Kcal and 45 to 60 gm of protein. It can be followed for a long periods.

Food Allowed

Refined cereals like rice, bread, biscuits, washed pulses, milk and milk products, egg and lean meats, starchy and low fibre vegetables, soft fruits, salt and sugar in moderation.

Mechanical Soft Diet

The mechanical soft diet is very close to the soft diet. It gets its name from the fact that household tools and machines, like a blender, meat grinder, or knife, are used to make foods easier to chew and swallow. In contrast to the soft diet, the mechanical soft diet does not restrict fat, fiber, spices, or seasonings. Only the texture and consistency of foods are changed. Fruits and vegetables may be soft-cooked or pureed. Meats, fish, and poultry can be cooked, ground, and moistened with sauce or gravy to make chewing and swallowing more comfortable. Breads and crackers may be limited at first, as they can be dry and difficult to swallow. The mechanical soft diet is appropriate for patients who are recovering from head, neck, or mouth surgery, who have dysphagia (difficulty swallowing), problem in the oesophagus (food tube), or who are too ill or weak to chew. The diet also benefits those who have poorly fitting dentures, no teeth, or other dental problems.

Review Questions

1. What is diet therapy? Write down its importance.
2. What are the main objectives of diet therapy?
3. Describe the therapeutic modifications of a normal diet.
4. What is the difference between enteral and parenteral feeding?
5. Write down a short note on full fluid diets.

Meal Planning and Food Exchange Lists

Introduction

The exchange lists were first published by a joint committee of the American Dietetics Association, American Diabetic Association and the US Public Health Services in 1950, and were revised in 1976.

Food exchange lists play an important role in diet planning. These lists are used in diet planning to make a quick and fairly accurate estimation of the nutritive value of diets. With the help of exchange lists, it becomes easy to estimate the fat, protein, and carbohydrate content of the meals. Along with these above written macronutrients various vitamins and minerals can also be calculated depending upon the need and suitability of person for whom diet is being planned.

The exchange list consists of commonly consumed food items that are categorized into 7 food groups. The grouping of foods is such that the carbohydrate, protein, fat and the calorie values are approximately equal for items listed under that group. One can use the exchange list to substitute or interchange items from a particular group to introduce variety in the meals.

The nutritive value of specific foods in the exchange list may slightly differ from the average value for that food exchange, but due to a variety of foods selected in the daily diet, these differences are cancelled out. So, any one food in particular food exchange list can be exchanged for any other food item in that list.

Food items from one group can be interchanged with another item from the same group however they cannot be interchanged with items listed under other groups.

Functions of Food Groups

Food Group

Body Building	Energy Giving	Protective
↓	↓	↓
Milk/Meat/Pulse	Cereal/Starch/Fat/Sugar	Vegetables [except starchy]/Fruits
↓	↓	↓
Protein	Carbohydrate & Fat	Minerals, Vitamins, Dietary Fibre

Weights and Measures Used

1 teaspoon (tsp) = 5 grams
1 tablespoon (tbsp) = 15 grams
1 small katori (SK) = 100 ml
1 medium katori (MK) = 150ml
1 big katori (BK) = 200ml
1 medium cup = 150ml
1 big cup = 200ml
1 medium glass = 240ml
1 big glass = 350ml

Each of the eight exchange lists have been discussed below:

Milk Exchange

1 cup of cow's milk provides protein content of 8g, which is taken as the constant for calculating this exchange. The milk products, which provide 8g of protein, are taken as one milk exchange.

On an average, each exchange of milk or milk product on this list contains 8g protein, 12g carbohydrate, 10g fat and 170 Kcal.

Nutritive composition of the comprehensive food exchange list

Food	Raw Food Amount (g)	Raw Food Measure (g)	Protein (g)	Carbohydrate (g)	Fat (g)	Energy (kcal)
Milk	250ml	1Cup	8	12	10	170
Meat	40	1egg	7	negligible	5	70
Pulse	30	3T	7	17	neg.	100
Cereal/starch	20/variable	1 bread slice	2	15	neg.	70
Vegetable A	100	1/2c	negligible	negligible	neg.	neg.
Vegetable B	variable	-	2	7	neg.	40
Fruit	variable	1portion	negligible	10	neg.	40
Fat	5	1t	-	-	5	45
Sugar	5	1t	-	5	-	20

Other food exchange lists are given in the appendix–4.

However, amount of fats varies on the type of milk, e.g., skim milk has only traces of fat while one exchange of buffalo's milk has 16g fat. If skim milk is substituted for cow's milk, 320ml of skim milk is taken as one milk exchange.

Meat Exchange

7 g of protein value is taken as constant in this exchange. The basis for this exchange is 40g of edible portion of mutton muscle providing 7g of protein. Each exchange of meat or meat substitute on this list provides on an average about 7g of protein, 5 g of fat, negligible carbohydrate and 70 kcal. In planning vegetarian diets, paneer or cheese can be conveniently utilized in the place of meat exchange as the milk carbohydrate (lactose) is lost while the preparation of these products. The amount of fat and energy content varies according to the kind of meat or meat substitute like fish, poultry etc. For example: when egg is used as one meat exchange, it is higher in fat and energy (7g fat and 90 kcal).

Pulse Exchange

The protein content of 7g is taken as the constant in this exchange i.e. that much portion of beans, pulses or their products, which provide 7 g of protein, is taken as one pulse exchange. The basis for this exchange is 30g of raw pulse containing 7g of protein. Each exchange of pulse on this list, except soybean, provides on an average about 7 g protein, 17 g carbohydrate, negligible fat and 100 kcal. One exchange of soybean (16g) provides more fat but lesser carbohydrate than the average pulse exchange. However, 30 g of raw pulses on sprouting weighs nearly 70 g due to water absorption. While sprouting, ascorbic acid, thiamine, riboflavin and niacin content of the pulses increase significantly.

Cereal/Starch Exchange

Each exchange of cereal provides on an average about 15 g carbohydrate, 2 g protein, negligible fat and 70 kcal. The basis of this exchange is one big slice of bread (30 g) or a small wheat flour chapatti made out of 20 g flour which contains about 15 g carbohydrate. The carbohydrate content of 15 g is taken as the constant in this exchange, i.e. that much portion of various cereal/starches and their products, which provides 15 g of carbohydrate, is taken as one cereal exchange. One cereal/starch exchange is about 20 g of almost all raw cereals or starches except root vegetables where 60 g makes one exchange because of their higher moisture content. Similarly, 30 g of bread is taken as one exchange.

Vegetable Exchange

The vegetable exchanges have been divided into two groups A and B on the basis of their carbohydrate content.

1) Vegetable A Exchange

This exchange includes leafy vegetables and the vegetables of the gourd family. All vegetables with 3 percent or less carbohydrate are included in this group. 100 g or ½ cup of vegetables make one exchange which has negligible fat and protein and provide about 12kcal.

Using only one exchange of vegetable A in the day's diet contributes negligible amount of protein, carbohydrate and fat, but if more than one exchange is used then their nutritive contribution is taken as:

2 exchanges of vegetable A = 1 exchange of vegetable B

2) Vegetable B Exchange

This exchange includes all the vegetables that are not included in the vegetable A exchange or cereal/starch exchange. A carbohydrate content of 7g is taken as the constant in this exchange, i.e. that much portion of various vegetables, which provide 7 g of carbohydrate, is taken as one vegetable B exchange. Each exchange of vegetable on this list provides on an average about 7 g carbohydrate, 2 g protein, negligible fat and 40 kcal although the amount of protein may vary slightly from 1 to 4 g. The weight/measure of one exchange of different vegetables in this exchange vary approximately from 50 to 200 g, depending upon whether they are high or low carbohydrate vegetables.

Like, tomato 194 g is taken as one exchange, since it is a low carbohydrate vegetable while for peas 44g is taken as one exchange, since it is a high carbohydrate vegetable.

Fruit Exchange

A portion of fruit that contains about 10 g of carbohydrate is taken as one fruit exchange. Here, the carbohydrate content of 10 g is taken as a constant for various fruits included in the fruit exchange. Each exchange of fruit on an average provides about 10 g of carbohydrate, negligible protein, fat and 40 kcal.

Like, if a low carbohydrate fruit such as musk melon or water melon is chosen, then 300 g is taken as high carbohydrate fruit such as dates or banana is chosen, then only 30 to 35 g constitutes one exchange while for moderate carbohydrate fruits like apple, apricot, cherries, guava, lichi, papaya, pear, plum etc, the amount varies from 75–100g per exchange.

Fat Exchange

Each fat exchange on this list provides about 5 g of fat and 45 kcal. Although some items such as nuts and oilseeds may also contain a small amount of protein and carbohydrate. Therefore, one exchange of nuts or oilseeds contains 2 g protein, 2 g carbohydrate, 60 kcal and 5 g of fat. In case of cream, then 25 g of it is taken as one fat exchange. One teaspoon or 5 g of fat or oil is the basis for this exchange. It means that much portion of various fats, oils, nuts and oil seeds, which provides 5 g fat, is taken as one fat exchange. It includes butter, edible fats and oils, such as hydrogenated fats and vegetables oils, creams, nuts, oilseeds, salad dressings etc.

Sugar Exchange

Each exchange on this list provides on an average 5 g carbohydrate and 20 kcal. One teaspoon or 5 g of sugar is the basis for this exchange. It means that much portion, which provides 5 g of carbohydrates, is taken as one sugar exchange. It includes sugar, jaggery, honey, jam, jellies, marmalades etc. When jams, jellies etc. are chosen then 7 to 8 g or 1 ½ teaspoon, is taken as 1 sugar exchange, as this amount of jam or jellies contains 5 g of carbohydrate. Food exchange lists are given in the appendix–1.

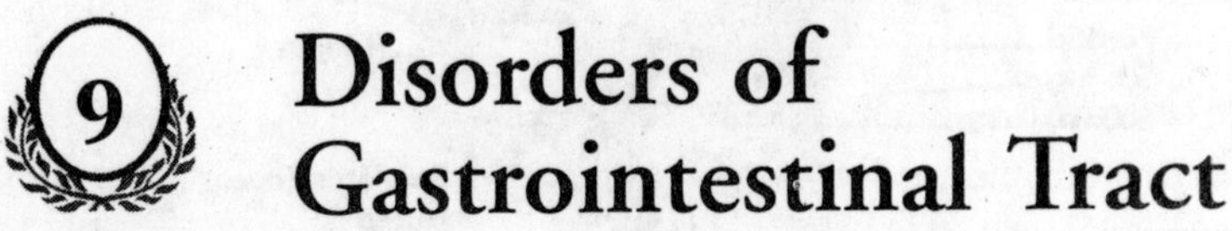

9 Disorders of Gastrointestinal Tract

Introduction

The gastrointestinal tract (GI tract), is also known as digestive tract, alimentary canal, or gut. It is involved in the digestion, absorption and utilization of food in the human body and expels out the remaining waste. The major functions of the GI tract are digestion and excretion.

Digestive system

The digestive system is the group of organs that breaks down food into chemical components that the body can absorb and use for energy and for building and repairing cells and tissues. The digestive system includes the salivary glands, oesophagus, stomach, pancreas, liver, biliary tract, small intestine and large intestine.

Chemical Digestion

Stomach

The stomach plays an important role in both chemical and mechanical digestion. Various chemicals in the stomach like the digestive enzymes interact to break down the food. In addition, hydrochloric acid creates suitable environment for the enzymes and assists in the digestion. Also, watery mucus provides a protective lining for the muscular walls of the stomach so it will not be digested

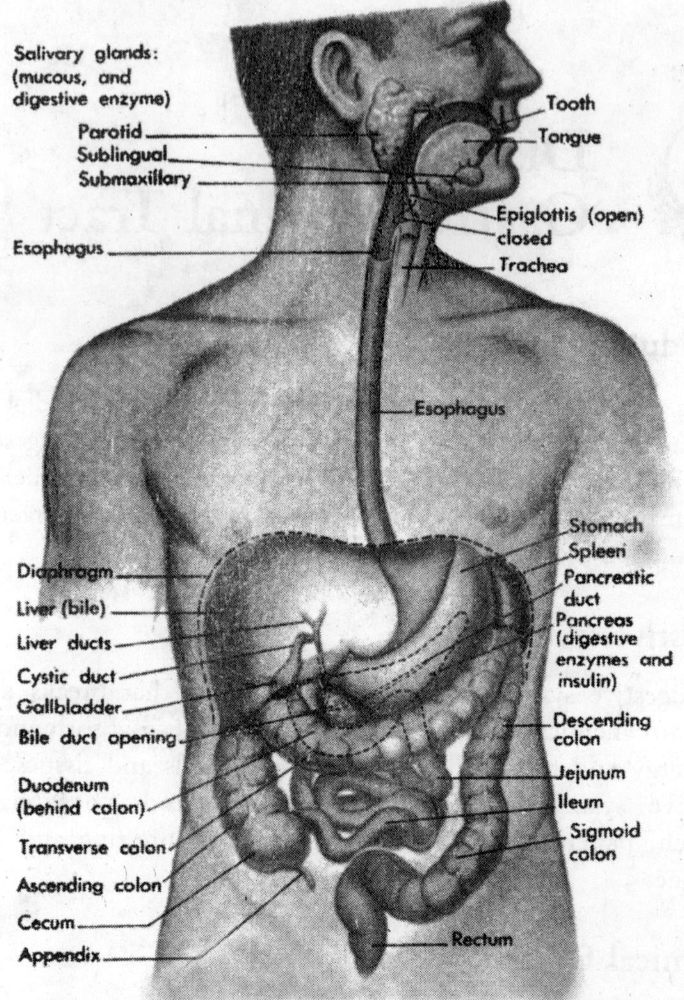

The Digestive System

Source: Kathleen M.L., Page-4

by the acid or enzymes. The mechanical action of the muscles in the stomach constrict and relax in a continuous motion blending, whipping, and stirring the stomach's contents into chyme, a pulpy substance that goes to the small intestine.

Small Intestine

The small intestine is the longest organ of the digestive tract. It is divided into three sections: the duodenum, the jejunum, and the ileum.

Duodenum

This is the place where the ultimate food digestion reaches its completion and where the acidity of chyme is nullified. The nutrients in the food are absorbed through the intestinal walls into the bloodstream. Carbohydrates are diminished into simpler sugars, proteins to amino acids, and fats to fatty acids and glycerol. Enzymes are secreted by the walls of the duodenum and unite with the bile (essential for the digestion and absorption of tenacious fatty materials) and pancreatic enzymes in the duodenum.

Jejunum

Peristalsis pushes the nutrient liquid out of the duodenum into the jejunum. A greater number of villi, microscopic, hair like structures, begin to absorb amino acids, sugars, fatty acids and glycerol from the digested contents of the small intestine. This part of the small intestine executes a digestive operation so that what is passed on to the large intestine is a thin watery substance almost completely devoid of nutrients.

Ileum

Ileum is the main part of the gastrointestinal tract, where absorption occurs. The greatest number of the estimated five or six million villi in the small intestine are found along the ileum.

The Liver, Gallbladder, and Pancreas

Digestive fluids from all these three meet at the common bile duct, and their movement is controlled by a sphincter muscle.

- The pancreas is a producer of digestive enzymes.
- The gallbladder is a small reservoir for bile.
- The liver reproduces nutrients so that they can be used for cell rebuilding and energy.

Various Enzymes and their Functions

Enzyme Origin	Enzyme	Nutrient Breaks Down	Product Of Enzyme Action	Place of Enzyme Action
Salivary glands	Salivary Amylase	Carbohydrates-sugars	Simple Sugars	Mouth
Gastric glands	Pepsin	Proteins	Amino Acids	Stomach
Liver	Bile	Fats/Lipids	Emulsified Fats	Small Intestine
Small intestine	Maltase, Lactase, Sucrase	Carbohydrates	Simple sugars	Small Intestine
Pancrease	Trypsin, Lipase, Amylase	Proteins, Fats/Lipids, Carbohydrates	Amino acids, Glycerol/ Fatty Acids, Simple Sugars	Small Intestine

Large Intestine

There are no villi in the large intestine and peristalsis is much less forceful than in the small intestine. As water is absorbed, the contents of the large intestine change from a watery liquid and are compressed into semisolid feces. Nerve endings in the large intestine signal the brain that it is time for a bowel movement. The fecal material moves through the colon down to several remaining inches known as the rectum and out through the anus an opening controlled by the outlet valves of the large intestine.

Mechanical Digestion

Mechanical digestion takes place in the mouth, where the saliva, teeth, and tongue all play an important role in the digestive process.

Saliva

The taste and smell of food send signals to the brain. The brain in turn sends messages to a system of salivary glands. Saliva is essentially made up of water and begins to soften up the food so it can pass more smoothly down the throat. Besides water there is ptyalin an enzyme who helps in the breakdown of the food into simpler forms.

Teeth

Teeth help to demolish chunks of food by a series of actions such as clamping, slashing, piercing, grinding and crushing. Teeth do the first drastic destruction to food in the digestive system.

Tongue

The surface of the tongue is covered in taste buds. The tongue consists of four types of taste buds—salty, sweet, sour, and bitter. It helps to remove, and dislocate food particles in the teeth and shifts food around in the mouth in order to assist in all the important acts of swallowing.

Peristalsis

Peristalsis is a series of synchronized, rhythmic muscle contractions. It is an automatic, vital process that propels food content through the gastrointestinal (GI) tract to facilitate normal digestion and the absorption of nutrients. Peristalsis is dependent upon the coordination between the muscles, nerves, and hormones in the digestive tract. Peristalsis helps a person to swallow, lying down or even standing on their head. It has another essential task besides assisting in the movement of food through the body.

Digestive Sphincters

The gastrointestinal tract is supplied with a number of muscular valves. These control and direct the quantity of food that goes through the digestive tract and inhibits the back movement of partially digested food.

Gastrointestinal disorders can be functional or organic in nature

Functional Disorders

Functional disorders are those in which the bowel looks normal but doesn't work properly. They are the most common problems affecting the colon and rectum, and include constipation, diarrhoea, irritable bowel syndrome (IBS) etc.

Organic Disorders

Organic disorders are those in which the anatomical structure of an organ is harmed to various degrees, thus interfering with its function like ulcers or cancer.

Constipation

Constipation is a decrease in the frequency of stool (the body's waste product) or difficulty in the formation or passage of stool. Constipation means that a person has three bowel movements or fewer in a week. The stool is hard and dry. Sometimes it is painful to pass. One may feel "draggy" and full. Prolonged bouts with constipation can lead to other health problems, such as haemorrhoids, varicose veins, indigestion, bad breath, headaches and body odor. This condition is truly universal and seen in all age groups, sex, socio-economic classes and races.

Types of Constipation

- Atonic constipation or lazy bowel (loss of muscle tone in the rectum).
- Spastic constipation (increase in the muscle tone which narrows the cavity).
- Obstructive constipation

Atonic Constipation

Atonic constipation is caused because of the sluggishness of the muscles of the intestine. Atonic constipation is due to the lack of adequate intake of fluids and lack of roughage in the diet. Irregular habits of the bowel movement and constant use of purgatives or enemas will result in loss of natural reflexes. It can also be due to fasting or avoiding foods containing unabsorbable cellulose in the form of vegetables and fruits. This leaves little residue for evacuation. Vitamin B deficiency and lack of potassium may also result in loss of bowel tone.

Spastic Constipation

Spastic constipation is brought about by a spasm or constriction of the muscles. Spastic constipation occurs due to irritating foods, irregular bowel movements, due to nervous disorders, excessive use of purgatives or mental stress.

Obstructive Constipation

Obstructive constipation is due to the obstruction of the large bowel or malignancy of the colon.

Causes and Risk Factors

Constipation is determined in the colon (large intestine), which is responsible for packaging and eliminating stool. As food moves

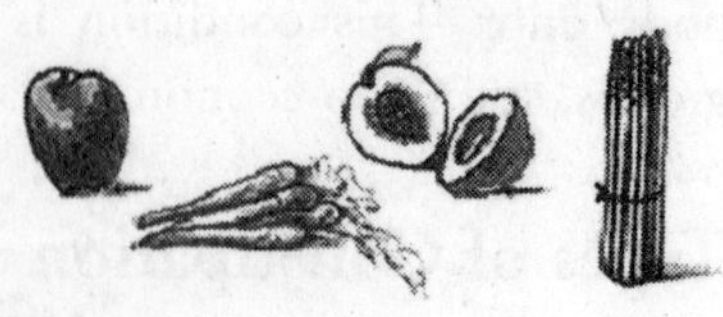

through the colon, it absorbs water while forming stool. Muscle contractions (squeezing motions) in the colon push the stool toward the rectum. By the time stool reaches the rectum, it is solid, because most of the water has been absorbed. The common causes of constipation are:

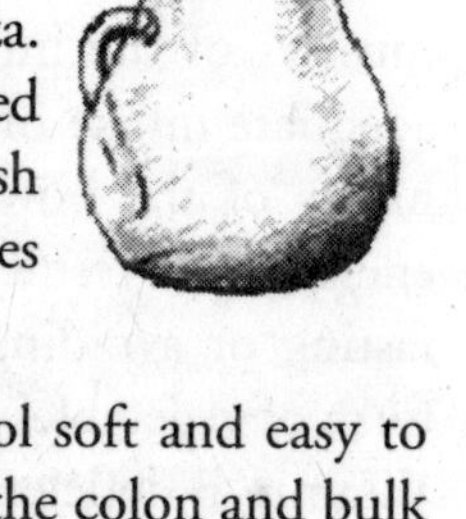

- *Less fibre in the diet*—Fibre helps form soft and bulky stools. It is found in many vegetables, fruits, and grains. Be sure to add fiber a little at a time, as sometimes more fibre can cause irritation and the body gets used to it slowly. Limit foods that have little or no fibre such as ice cream, cheese, meat, snacks like chips and pizza. Examples of fibre-rich foods are unprocessed wheat bran, unrefined breakfast cereals, fresh fruits (except bananas), dried fruits, vegetables (except potatoes), grainy breads and legumes.
- *Not enough liquid*—Liquid helps keep the stool soft and easy to pass. Liquids like water and juice add fluid to the colon and bulk to stools, making movements softer and easier to pass. Drink plenty of water and other liquids such as fruit and vegetable juices and clear soups. Try not to drink liquids that contain caffeine or alcohol. As the caffeine and alcohol tend to dry out the digestive system. Recommended daily consumption of liquid is eight to ten glasses per day.
- *Lack of exercise*—Regular exercise helps the digestive system stay active and healthy. Lack of exercise makes the digestive system sluggish.
- *Medications*—Some medications can also cause constipation. They include calcium pills, pain pills with codeine in them, some antacids, iron pills, diuretics, and medicines for depression
- *Irritable bowel syndrome (IBS)* is a common disorder of the intestines that leads to crampy pain, gassiness, bloating, and

changes in bowel habits. Some people with IBS may develop constipation.

- *Pregnancy* also leads to constipation. During pregnancy, the body produces more female hormones than normal. It is the job of these hormones to make sure that the pregnancy develops normally. But they also automatically slow down the woman's intestinal movements. One of these hormones, called progesterone, acts by relaxing muscle. Many women take iron supplements during pregnancy, which can also be a contributing factor to constipation. And the last reason is that the growing baby puts pressure on the bowel, while the discomfort of its weight and general tiredness may lead to a lack of exercise, both can slow down bowel movements.
- *Lifestyle changes*, such as aging and traveling can also cause constipation.
- *Excessive use of laxatives* can cause laxative abuse—A laxative is a food or chemical substance that acts to loosen the bowels by softening and increasing the bulk of bowel contents, increasing the amount of water in the colon and lubricating the intestinal walls. Over time, laxatives can damage nerve cells in the colon and interfere with the colon's natural ability to contract.
- *Ignoring the urge to have a bowel movement.* One should always give enough time to have a bowel movement.
- *Diseases such as multiple sclerosis*, Parkinson's disease, stroke, spinal cord injuries, diabetes, under-active and over-active thyroid gland, uremia (excess urine waste product), colorectal cancer, depression, colon tumors, diverticulosis and Hirschsprung's disease also cause constipation.

Symptoms

Depending on diet, age and daily activities, regular bowel movements can mean anything from three bowel movements per day to one every three days. If someone experiences hard, compacted stools that are difficult or painful to pass, the urge to move the bowels, or no bowel movement over three days for adults and four days for children, the person may have constipation. The symptoms of constipation are as follows:

- Headache
- Coated tongue
- Fowl breath
- Lack of appetite
- Feeling sluggish
- Abdominal swelling
- Abdominal bloating
- Nausea

Dietary Management during Constipation

Usually there is no special diet for constipation. In a normal regular diet, modifications in fibre and fluid intake are made.

Fibre

Fibre increases the motility of the small intestine and colon. A high fibre intake prevents or relieves constipation but the amount of fibre required for this effect varies considerably from individual to individual.

Fluid

Around 12 to 14 glasses of water are suggested. Along with water, soups and broths should always be given.

Diarrhoea

Diarrhoea is a very common symptom with many possible causes. The term is used to describe an increase in frequency of bowel motions, increased stool liquidity or sometimes a sense of faecal urgency. Actual definition of diarrhoea is "the passage of greater

High-Fibre Foods

Fruit/Vegetables			Breads/Cereals
Apples raw			Black-eyed peas, cooked
Peaches,	Broccoli,	raw	Kidney beans, cooked
Raspberries	Brussels sprouts,	raw	Lima beans, cooked
	Cabbage,	raw	Whole-grain cereal, cold
	Carrots,	raw	(All-Bran, Total, Bran Flakes)
	Cauliflower,	raw	Whole-grain cereal, hot
	Spinach,	cooked	(oatmeal,) Whole-wheat

than 300 ml of liquid faeces in 24 hours". Diarrhea occurs when insufficient fluid is absorbed by the colon. As part of the digestion process, or due to fluid intake, food is mixed with large amounts of water. Thus, digested food is essentially liquid prior to reaching the colon. The colon absorbs water, leaving the remaining material as a semisolid stool. If the colon is damaged or inflamed, however, absorption is inhibited, and watery stools result. Almost everyone has diarrhea at some point in his or her life. In developing countries, where illnesses that cause diarrhea are more common and where healthcare is less readily available, diarrhea is a major health concern because of its potential to cause severe, life-threatening dehydration. Infants and the elderly are more prone to dehydration from diarrhea.

Causes of Diarrhoea

The causes of diarrhoea have been divided into external and internal factors.

External Factors

a) **Infection**—usually comes from the source of contaminated food/water. These types of diarrhoea are often contagious. The common infective agents are

- Bacteria—E. coli, Salmonella, Shigella, Campylobacter, etc.

- Parasites—Entamoeba histolytica, Giardia Lamblia, Cryptosporidium, worms, etc.
- Virus—Rotavirus, Norwalk virus, etc.

b) **Foods**—Spicy, hot food can cause diarrhoea.

c) **Toxins**—Chemicals, decayed food or poison can cause diarrhoea.

d) **Mechanical**—Ingestion of any hard food substance can also cause diarrhoea.

e) **Habits**—Overindulgence in alcohol and irregular dietary habit can also cause diarrhoea.

f) **Drugs and Therapy**—Long-term use of laxatives, antacids, cancer drugs, antibiotics, radiation therapy, etc., can produce chronic diarrhoea.

Internal Factors

a) **Mind and Neurological**—anxiety, worries, excessive thinking and tension often cause vagal stimulation. This stimulation causes more acid secretion in the stomach, which often induces diarrhoea. Also, some women often suffer from diarrhoea during menses, since the rectum becomes irritable from adjacent menstruating uterus.

b) **Deficiency**—Vitamins, minerals specially zinc.

c) **Diseases**—Cancer, tuberculosis, AIDS, crohn's disease, ulcerative colitis, irritable bowel syndrome (IBS), liver diseases, typhoid, etc.

d) **Allergies**—Food allergy, lactose intolerance, mal-absorption, etc.

Types of Diarrhoea

Diarrhoea can be classified as acute and chronic depending upon the period of suffering and seriousness. Usually, acute diarrhoea occurs suddenly and lasts for a few days at the most, whereas chronic diarrhoea is persistent and lasts longer (more than 10 days) with serious inflammatory/irritable bowel diseases.

- Acute Watery (passage of loose or watery stool without visible blood)
- Dysentery (diarrhoea with visible blood and mucus)
- Chronic Diarrhoea (due to non-infectious causes such as sensitivity to gluten or lactose or inherited metabolic disorders).

Physiological Disturbances in the Body

- Painful abdominal cramps and vomiting,
- Weak pulse.
- Fall in blood pressure.
- Urine quantity and frequency falls.
- Dehydration impairs the skin elasticity.

Treatment of Acute Diarrhoea

In sanitary living conditions, with ample food and water available, an otherwise healthy patient typically recovers from the common viral infections in a few days and at most a week. However, for ill or malnourished individuals diarrhea can lead to severe dehydration and can become life-threatening without treatment.

Diarrhoea can also be a symptom of more serious diseases, such as dysentery, cholera, or botulism, and can also be a indicative of a chronic syndrome such as crohn's disease. Diarrhoea can also be caused by dairy intake in those who are lactose intolerant.

- Symptomatic treatment for diarrhea involves the patient consuming adequate amounts of water to replace that loss, preferably mixed with electrolytes to provide essential salts and some amount of nutrients. For many people, further treatment is unnecessary. Usually the ORS (oral rehydration salts) are given.

Composition of ORS	
Sodium chloride	3.5g
Potassium chloride	1.5g
Sodium bicarbonate	2.5g
Glucose	20g
To be dissolved in one litre of potable water	

Dietary Management in Diarrhoea

The objectives of dietary treatment in chronic diarrhoea are:

1. To meet the nutritional requirements.
2. To correct electrolyte losses and water.

Energy—Increased by 10 to 20 percent.

Protein—Increased by 40 to 45 percent.

Carbohydrates—To meet increased energy needs.

Fats—Intake is restricted to 15 to 20 percent.

Many things can cause diarrhoea including diet and medications. Take special care to:

- Drink at least 8 to 10 glasses of fluid everyday. This will replace lost fluids. Water, juices (except prune juice), broth, ginger ale, and weak tea are all good sources of fluid.
- The treatment of diarrhea is different for each individual.
- One should limit foods that contain caffeine such as coffee, strong tea and aerated beverages.
- In some cases milk and milk products such as milk, cheese, pudding and ice cream can made diarrhea worse. Lactose-free milk or soy beverages may be better tolerated.
- Limit use of high fat foods such as fried foods, fatty meats, high fat desserts, excess butter, margarine, higher fat milk products and greasy snack foods

- Reduce the amount of fibre in the diet. Fibre is found mostly in fruits, vegetables, whole grain breads and cereals, nuts and seeds. Try a low fiber diet.
- Try eating several small meals throughout the day.
- Limit use of dried fruits, berries, rhubarb, legumes (lentils, kidney beans, lima beans), peas, corn, broccoli, spinach and nuts. They may make diarrhea worse for some people.
- If someone has a gas or cramping problem. Then he should avoid foods that can increase gas production. These include dried peas and beans, broccoli, cabbage, cauliflower, onions, brussels sprouts, carbonated beverages, beer and chewing gum.

Foods to avoid

- High sugar
- Alcohol
- Lactose
- High protein diet
- Fats and oils
- Processed food like maida

Crohn's Disease and Ulcerative Colitis

Crohn's disease causes inflammation in the small intestine. Crohn's disease usually occurs in the lower part of the small intestine, called the ileum, but it can affect any part of the digestive tract, from the mouth to the anus. The inflammation extends deep into the lining of the affected organ. The inflammation can cause pain and can make the intestines empty frequently, resulting in diarrhea. Ulcerative colitis and Crohn's disease are usually same. *The only difference is that ulcerative colitis involves only top layer of lining of large intestine where as in crohn's disease all layers of intestine may be involved.*

When the inflammation occurs in the rectum and lower part of the colon it is called ulcerative proctitis. If the entire colon is affected it is called pan colitis. If only the left side of the colon is affected it is called limited or distal colitis.

Symptoms

a) Mild Cases

- Abdominal pain and cramping.
- Bloody diarrhoea.
- Pain is felt in the area of the navel or on the right side.
- Ulcers.
- Lack of appetite and weight loss.

b) Severe cases

- Fever
- Fatigue
- Problems outside the digestive tract including arthritis, eye inflammation, skin disorders, inflammation of liver and bile ducts.

Gastritis

Gastritis is an inflammation of the lining of the stomach.

Signs and Symptoms

- Abdominal cramping and pain,
- Nausea
- Vomiting
- Diarrhoea
- Fever
- Loss of appetite

- Belching or gas
- Weakness

Causes

- Bacterial or viral infection (infection by a virus is contagious).
- Excess stomach acid caused by heavy smoking, alcohol use, caffeine, improper diet such as spicy, greasy foods.
- Use of drugs such as Aspirin, non-steroidal anti-inflammatories, cortisone.
- Stress.

Preventive Measures

- Eat regularly and moderately.
- Stop smoking.
- Limit or avoid alcohol and caffeine.
- Avoid foods that don't digest easily.
- Don't eat solid foods on the first day of the attack, give stomach rest and drink liquids only, milk or water are preferred. Add bland foods to the diet slowly. Avoid greasy, spicy foods.

Other important Gastrointestinal Disorders are

Irritable Bowel Syndrome (IBS)

Irritable bowel syndrome (also called spastic colon, irritable colon, or nervous stomach) is a condition in which the colon muscle contracts more readily than in people without IBS. A number of factors can trigger IBS including certain foods, medicines, and emotional stress. Symptoms of IBS include abdominal pain and cramps, excess gas, bloating, and a change in bowel habits such as harder, looser, or more urgent stools than normal. Often people with IBS have alternating constipation and diarrhea.

Treatment includes avoiding caffeine, increasing fiber in the diet, drinking more fluids, monitoring which foods trigger IBS (and avoiding these foods), quitting smoking, minimizing stress or learning different ways to cope with stress, and sometimes taking medicines as prescribed by the doctor.

Haemorrhoids

Haemorrhoids, also known as "piles," are enlarged veins located in the lower rectum or anus that are caused by blood blockage in the veins of the haemorrhoidal complex. The haemorrhoids begin above the internal opening of the anus and may become large enough to protrude. The subsequent squeezing of them while sitting brings on pain. Hardened stools, or constipation, is one of the primary causes of haemorrhoids.

Anal Fissures

Anal fissures are splits or cracks in the lining of the anal opening. The most common cause of an anal fissure is the passage of very hard or watery stools. The crack in the anal lining exposes the underlying muscles that control the passage of stool through the anus and out of the body. An anal fissure is one of the most painful problems because the exposed muscles become irritated from exposure to stool or air, and leads to intense burning pain, bleeding, or spasm after bowel movements.

Initial treatment for anal fissures includes pain medicine, dietary fiber to reduce the occurrence of large, bulky stools, and sitz baths (sitting in a few inches of warm water). If these treatments don't relieve pain, surgery might be needed to decrease spasm in the sphincter muscle.

Perianal Abscesses

Perianal abscesses can occur when the tiny anal glands that open on the inside of the anus become blocked, and the bacteria always present in these glands cause an infection. When pus develops, an abscess forms. Treatment includes draining the abscess, usually under local anesthesia.

Diverticular Disease

Diverticulosis is the presence of small outpouchings (diverticula) in the muscular wall of the large intestine that form in weakened areas of the bowel. They usually occur in the sigmoid colon, the high-pressure area of the lower large intestine.

Diverticular disease is very common and occurs in 10 percent of people over age 40 and in 50 percent of people over age 60 in western cultures. It is often caused by too little roughage (fibre) in the diet. Diverticulosis rarely causes symptoms but when it occurs, they might include tenderness over the affected area or muscle spasms in the abdomen.

Laxative

Laxative is a drug or other substance used to stimulate the action of the intestines in eliminating waste from the body. The term **laxative** usually refers to a mild-acting substance, whereas, the substances of increasingly drastic action are known as **cathartics**, **purgatives**, and **hydrogogues**, respectively. Laxatives or cathartics fall into three general categories: irritants that stimulate the muscular action of the intestines, compounds that increase the amount of bulk in the intestines either by withdrawing water from the body or by increasing the bulk when combined with fluids, and lubricants such as mineral oil, which ease the passage of waste and counteract excessive drying of the intestinal contents. Frequent or regular use of cathartics may seriously disrupt the **natural digestive processes**. When food and even waste products are forced out of the intestinal tract too rapidly, the body is deprived of vital substances, including the nutrients absorbed in the small intestine and the water, vitamins, and minerals extracted from the waste matter in the large intestine. Vitamins A and D, which are soluble in oil, are removed from the body even when the least irritating laxative, mineral oil, is taken. Laxatives should be avoided especially when there is abdominal pain. An inflamed appendix may rupture after the use of a laxative.

Complications of diverticular disease happen in about 10 percent of people with outpouchings. They include infection or inflammation (diverticulitis), bleeding, and obstruction. Treatment includes antibiotics, increased fluids, and a special diet. Surgery is needed in about half the patients who have complications to remove the involved segment of the colon.

Review Questions

1. What is constipation? How can we cure it?
2. Write down the dietary management of constipation.
3. How does diarrhoea affect our body system? Give its dietary management.
4. What points should be kept in mind while planning diet for a patient suffering from diarrhoea?
5. What are laxatives? Should we consume them on daily basis?

10 Disorders of Cardiovascular System

Introduction

Cardiovascular diseases refer to the class of diseases that involve the heart and the blood vessels (arteries and veins). While the term clinically refers to any disease that affects the cardiovascular system. Heart diseases affect people of all ages. The blood vessels within the heart, leaving the heart or the heart valves may be diseased. A heart attack and a stroke by no means are always fatal. Some can go back to their old activities, some remain invalid and some are handicapped. Coronary artery diseases (CAD) are highly predictable, preventable and treatable.

Physiology of Heart

The heart is located in the chest between the lungs behind the sternum and above the diaphragm. It is surrounded by the pericardium. Its size is about that of a fist, and its weight is about 250–300 g. Located above the heart are the great vessels: the superior and inferior vena cava, the pulmonary artery and vein, as well as the aorta. The aortic arch lies behind the heart.

The walls of the heart are composed of cardiac muscle, called myocardium. It also has striations similar to skeletal muscle. It consists of four compartments: the right and left atria and ventricles. The left ventricular free wall and the septum are much thicker than the right ventricular wall. This is logical since the left ventricle pumps blood to the systemic circulation, where the pressure is considerably higher than for the pulmonary circulation, which arises from right ventricular outflow.

The heart has four valves. Between the right atrium and ventricle lies the tricuspid valve, and between the left atrium and ventricle is the mitral valve. The pulmonary valve lies between the right ventricle and the pulmonary artery, while the aortic valve lies in the outflow tract of the left ventricle (controlling flow to the aorta).

The blood returns from the systemic circulation to the right atrium and from there goes through the tricuspid valve to the right ventricle. It is ejected from the right ventricle through the pulmonary valve to the lungs. Oxygenated blood returns from the lungs to the left atrium, and from there through the mitral valve to the left ventricle. Finally blood is pumped through the aortic valve to the aorta and the systemic circulation.

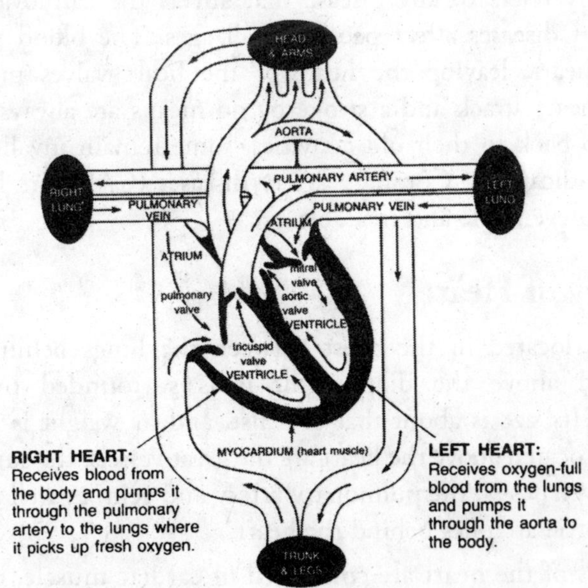

Structure of heart Pump

Source: Kathleen M.L., Page-738

Causes of Cardiovascular Diseases

a) Cholesterol

Cholesterol is a naturally occurring fat, which is fundamentally required for good health. It is the precursor to both the male hormone testosterone and the female hormone estrogen, which cannot be made without it. In addition, it performs other vital functions in the body. In most people, the levels of cholesterol found in the blood have little or nothing to do with fats consumed in the diet.

- Cholesterol is a complex, fatty substance, which is produced by the liver, and the body needs cholesterol to function normally.
- Cholesterol is also found in some foods such as organ meats (i.e. liver, kidneys, brain), seafood and egg yolks.
- Diet only accounts for 20 percent of the cholesterol in body with the remaining 80 percent produced by the liver.
- Cholesterol is present in cell walls or membranes everywhere in the body, including the brain, nerves, muscles, skin, liver, intestines and heart.
- The body uses it to produce many hormones and parts of the cells. In fact, without cholesterol, body cannot function.
- The problem occurs when there is too much cholesterol in the bloodstream, the extra amount is deposited in arteries, including the coronary arteries, where it leads to the narrowing and blockages that are responsible for the heart diseases.

Cholesterol Levels (mg/dl)	
High	240 or more
Borderline-high	200-239
Desirable	Below 200

b) Lipoproteins

Lipoproteins play an important role in the transportation of cholesterol and other fats across approximately 260,000 kilometers of blood vessels, arteries and capillaries to various body tissues to be used, stored or excreted. There are several types of lipoproteins. Here are the most important ones to monitor for heart health. Some of the important are as follows:

Low-Density Lipoproteins (LDL)

- LDL molecules carry cholesterol from the liver to other parts of the body. Cholesterol carried by these molecules (LDL cholesterol) is called "bad" cholesterol because it can lead to a buildup of plaque in the lining of the arteries. This can reduce blood flow, and may lead to the artery being fully blocked, which in turn can lead to a heart attack or stroke. Therefore, one should always keep check on the LDL ("bad") cholesterol in the blood.

LDL Levels (mg/dl)	
High	160 or above
Borderline	130-159
Desirable	100-129
Desirable for people with heart disease	Below 100

The Lipid profile does not measure (LDL) level directly but instead estimates it with the help of *Friedewald* equation using levels of other cholesterol such as HDL.

LDL cholesterol = total cholesterol–HDL cholesterol–(0.20 x triglycerides) (In mg/dl)

High-Density Lipoproteins (HDL)

- HDL molecules gather up extra cholesterol from around the body and carry it back to the liver, where it is broken down. Cholesterol carried by these molecules (HDL cholesterol) is called "good cholesterol" because it doesn't block the blood vessels.

HDL Levels (mg/dl)	
Low	Below 40
Intermediate	40-59
High	60 or more

c) Triglycerides

- High levels of triglycerides (another fatty substance found in the blood) have been linked to low levels of HDL cholesterol, obesity and diabetes, which are all risk factors for heart disease. Triglycerides can be converted to LDL cholesterol in the liver.

Triglyceride Levels (mg/dl)	
Very High	1000
High	400-1000
Borderline	200-399
Normal	Below 200

A high LDL cholesterol level means that an individual has more cholesterol in the blood than the body needs. The higher the LDL cholesterol level, the greater the risk of developing coronary heart diseases. Anyone can develop high LDL cholesterol, no matter what his or her age, weight, gender, race or ethnic background. High cholesterol has no warning signs. One can lower LDL cholesterol and significantly bring down the risk of heart disease.

d) Trans Fatty Acids

Trans fatty acids have been found to raise lipoproteins levels, thus raising the risk of coronary heart disease. They raise LDL cholesterol and lower HDL cholesterol. Trans fatty acids are more atherogenic. Trans fatty acids in the diet come from two main sources:

1) **Bacterial Fermentation**—In the gut of ruminants, Trans fatty acids are produced. Meat and dairy products contain trans fatty acids.

2) **Hydrogenated Fats**—Hydrogenation of vegetable oils leads to production of trans fatty acids depending upon the degree of hydrogenation. The amount of trans fatty acids in food products can vary from 5 to 40per cent.

Cardiovascular Disorders mainly include

- Hypertension
- Atherosclerosis
- Myocardial infarction
- Congestive heart failure

Cardiovascular disease usually occurs as a result of arterial damage. The symptoms and treatments depend on a particular set of arteries that have been affected. In coronary heart disease, atherosclerotic plaques (inflamed fatty deposits in the blood vessel wall) obstruct the coronary arteries. Narrowing of arteries is called arterial stenosis. When the blockages become severe enough, the blood flow to the heart is restricted (cardiac ischemia), especially during increased demand like during exertion or emotion and this results in angina pectoris. The acute stage of coronary heart disease occurs when one of the plaque ruptures, forming a thrombus (blood clot) that acutely occludes the whole artery. The portion of the heart muscle supplied by that artery dies, leading to myocardial infarction. This may result in the death of the patient if the affected area is large enough. If the patient survives, congestive heart failure may result. Similarly, inflammation and blood clots may obstruct the cerebral arteries, those supplying the brain. As the disease progresses, an artery may be transiently blocked, causing cerebral ischemia. This results in a transient ischemic attack , called a mini-stroke. If the obstruction is severe, a cerebrovascular accident, or stroke may result, due to the death of brain tissue supplied by the artery.

The high socio-economic group people adopt an adverse lifestyle such as high-saturated fatty acids diet, sedentary lifestyle and cigarette smoking. Thus the chances of coronary heart diseases increase.

Common Symptoms of Heart Diseases

Chest pain is the most common symptom and is often described as a sensation of tightness, pressure, or squeezing. Pain radiates most often to the left arm, but may also radiate to the jaw, neck, right arm, back, and epigastrium. Some of the other important symptoms are:

- Discomfort
- Sweating
- Weakness
- Nausea
- Vomiting
- Arrhythmia
- Loss of consciousness

Often a combination of several different problems cause heart problems, which include the following:

- Weakened heart muscle
- Damaged heart valves.
- Blocked blood vessels supplying the heart muscle (coronary arteries), leading to a heart attack.
- Toxic exposures, like alcohol or cocaine.
- Infections.
- High blood pressure that results in thickening of the heart muscle (left ventricular hypertrophy).
- Pericardial disease, such as a large collection of fluid around the heart in the space between the heart muscle and the thick layer of pericardium surrounding the heart and/or a thickened pericardium, which does not allow the heart to work properly.
- Congenital heart diseases.
- Prolonged, serious arrhythmias.

Risk Factors

There are so many factors which lead to heart problems. Many of the important risk factors are given below:

Advanced Age

With ageing, the chances of heart diseases increase. It has been found that approximately 65 percent of all heart attacks and 85 percent of all coronary heart disease (CHD) deaths occur to people aged 65 or older. CHD is the leading cause of death for people over 65 years of age. In short, coronary heart disease's risk increases with age.

Sex

All throughout life, men have a much higher risk of death from CHD than do women. Major increases in the occurrence of heart disease begin for men at the age of 35. Women begin to display a marked increase after menopause.

Diabetes

Heart diseases often go hand-in-hand with diabetes. Persons with diabetes are at a much greater risk for heart attacks. Serious cardiovascular disease can begin before the age of 30 in persons with diabetes. Damage to the coronary arteries is two to four times more likely in asymptomatic persons with diabetes than in the general population.

Dyslipidemia (elevated serum cholesterol or triglyceride levels)

- High serum concentration of low density lipoprotein (LDL, "bad cholesterol")
- Low serum concentration of functioning high density lipoprotein (HDL, "good cholesterol") particles.

Tobacco Smoking

Smoking is the single largest contributor to the risk of having a heart attack. In fact, smokers are twice as likely to have a heart attack than are non smokers, and they are between 2 and 4 times more likely to experience sudden death. Exposure to environmental tobacco smoke in the home and at the workplace has also been shown to increase the risk for CHD. Yet the ability to recover from tobacco use is quite remarkable. Within three years after quitting, the risk of death from heart disease for people who smoke a pack, a day or less is almost the same as for people who never smoked.

High Blood Pressure

High blood pressure increases the heart's workload, causing it to enlarge and weaken. It increases the risk for a number of diseases, including congestive heart failure, kidney failure, heart attack, and stroke. When other risk factors are present, the risk from high blood pressure increases several times over. High blood pressure can be controlled through proper diet, losing excess weight, regular exercise, restricting salt intake, and through the use of antihypertensive medications.

Obesity

Obesity (in particular central obesity, also referred to as abdominal or male-type obesity). Excessive body weight has been shown to correlate with various diseases, particularly cardiovascular diseases.

A Sedentary Life Style

A sedentary life style or physical inactivity plays a significant role in the occurrence of heart disease. It has been recommended for the people of all ages to include a minimum of 30 minutes of physical activity of moderate intensity such as brisk walking on alternate, if not all, days of the week. Examples of such activities include aerobics, jogging, and vigorous walking. As a rule of thumb, any exercise that makes an individual breath hard and heartbeat rapidly should provide this benefit. Recent studies have indicated that even modest levels of low-intensity exercise will provide increased cardiovascular fitness. These activities include walking for pleasure, gardening, housework, and dancing. It is also acknowledged that for most people, greater health benefits can be obtained by engaging in physical activity of more vigorous intensity or of longer duration.

Elevated Serum Levels of Homocysteine

Homocysteine is made from protein in the body. The amino acid methionine is converted into homocysteine in the body but vitamin

B6, B12 and folic acid should be present in adequate amount. A high level of blood serum homocysteine is considered to be a marker of potential cardiovascular (risk factor for heart attack and stroke) disease.

Stress or Clinical Depression

Stress does contribute to heart disease in certain individuals. It leads to high blood pressure, high cholesterol, and other cardiac risk factors (e.g. smoking, overweight, etc.) in many individuals.

Hypothyroidism (a Slow-Acting Thyroid)

The cardiovascular risk in people with hypothyroidism is related to an increased risk of functional cardiovascular abnormalities and to an increased risk of atherosclerosis. It has been found that a lesser degree of thyroid hormone deficiency may affect the cardiovascular system. Hypothyroid patients, even those with subclinical hypothyroidism, have impaired endothelial function, normal/depressed systolic function, left ventricular diastolic dysfunction at rest, and systolic and diastolic dysfunction on effort, which may result in poor physical exercise capacity. There is also a tendency to increase diastolic blood pressure.

Hypertension

Blood pressure is the pressure of blood in the arteries and it is the force exerted by the bloodstream on the artery walls. The higher

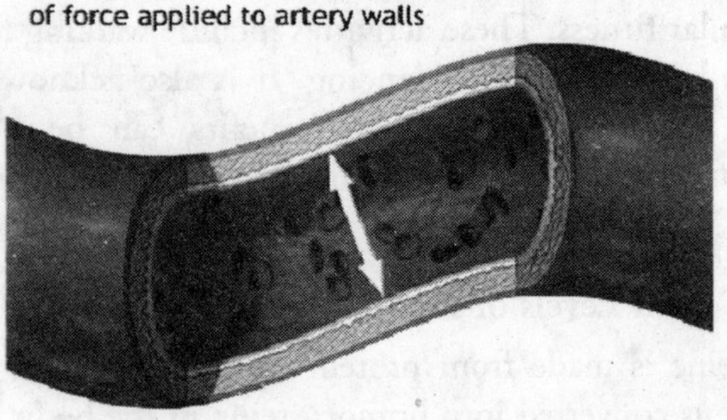

WHO Classification of Blood Pressure	
Normotension	SBP ≤ 140mm of Hg and DBP ≤ 90mm of Hg
Borderline hypertension	SBP 141 to 159mm of Hg and DBP 91 to 94 mm of Hg
Hypertension	SBP ≥ 160 mm of Hg and DBP ≥ 95 mm of Hg

the blood pressure, the greater the risk of developing narrowed arteries, which can lead to heart problems, kidney disease and stroke. Hypertension is defined as sustained elevated arterial blood pressure exceeding 140 over 90 mm Hg (a systolic pressure above 140 with a diastolic pressure above 90).

Systolic Blood Pressure (SBP) is consistently over 140 (systolic is the "top" number of blood pressure measurement, which represents the pressure generated when the heart beats).

Diastolic Blood Pressure (DBP) is consistently over 90 (diastolic is the "bottom" number of blood pressure measurement, which represents the pressure in the vessels when the heart is at rest).

Hypertension can involve many organs and systems including endocrine glands, kidneys, central nervous system and autonomic nervous system. It has been clearly shown to increase the risk of developing stroke, coronary heart disease, congestive heart failure, peripheral vascular disease. The risk of hypertension increases with blood pressure level. More than 90 percent of people with hypertension have no identifiable cause of elevated blood pressure and are said to have primary, essential, idiopathic and rest of the people, with identifiable cause of hypertension are said to have secondary hypertension.

The secondary hypertension may be due to:

- Renal diseases
- Use of oral contraceptives in case of the women
- Endocrine diseases such as hyperthyroidism

Causes and Risk Factors of Hypertension

Obesity

The relationship between obesity and hypertension appears to be linear and exists throughout the non-obese range. But the strength of the association of obesity with hypertension varies among different racial and ethnic groups.

Age and Sex

Systolic blood pressure rises steeply from infancy to adulthood and then levels off. Diastolic blood pressure on the other hand rises approximately 10mm between the ages of 20 to 60 and gradually declines after that. Higher prevalence of hypertension has been found among males from adolescence till 45 years of age. After this age mean blood pressure values are higher in women.

Heredity

Heredity is also associated with hypertension.

Exercise and Activity

Increased physical activity and exercise have the long-term hypotensive effect.

Dietary Factors

A variety of physiological mechanisms some of which may be influenced by diet can contribute to hypertension. Some of the dietary factors, such as total energy, dietary fat, dietary fiber, sodium, potassium, and alcohol have been linked to the blood pressure.

Volume of Water in the Body

Hypertension is very often a result of the body adjusting to blood volume loss. The most common cause of lower blood volume is dehydration. Since blood is more than 83 percent water, the level of available water in the body heavily affects its total volume. When the body detects a loss of blood volume, it closes off less active capillary beds in order to maintain proper blood flow to the more active areas.

These vessel closings cause a rise in tension inside the muscle mass, which is known as "hypertension." More water allows for proper blood volume and less tension. Hypertension, more commonly known as high blood pressure, is an adaptive process to a gross body water deficiency.

Condition of the Kidneys

If the blood vessels in the kidneys are damaged, they may stop removing wastes and extra fluid from the body. The extra fluid in the blood vessels may then raise blood pressure even more.

Condition of Blood Vessels

The condition of blood vessels is directly related to the hypertension.

Levels of Various Hormones in the Body

Epinephrine, norepinephrine, aldosterone, corticosteroids and thyroid hormones affect the hypertension. Aldosterone increases the sodium ion absorption in the distal convoluted tubules of the kidneys.

Tyramine is derived from the amino acid tyrosine. When, the foods high in tyramine are ingested, hypertension can result. A large dietary intake of tyramine can cause the '**tyramine pressor response**,' which is defined as an systolic blood pressure of 30 mm Hg or more.

Symptoms

- Blood in urine
- Nose bleed
- Irregular heartbeat
- Ear noise or buzzing
- Tiredness

- Confusion
- Vision changes
- Angina-like chest pain
- Heart failure

Complications

- Heart attacks
- Congestive heart failure
- Blood vessel damage
- Kidney damage or Brain damage
- Loss of vision

Prevention

- Exercise to help the heart
- Adjust the diet as needed
- Keep the blood pressure checked at regular intervals

Tips to Lower Salt Intake

- Look for foods that are labeled "low-sodium," "sodium-free," "no salt added," or "unsalted." Check the total sodium content on food labels.
- Don't cook with salt or add salt to food. Try pepper, garlic, lemon, or other spices for flavor instead.
- Avoid foods that are naturally high in sodium, like meats (particularly cured meats, bacon, hot dogs, sausage, ham, and salami), nuts, olives, pickles, soy and worcestershire sauces, tomato and other vegetable juices, and cheese.

Energy—Hypocaloric diet is recommended.

Protein—Excess amount of animal protein should be avoided.

Fat—Low fat diets i.e. about 20 percent of energy should come from fats. More of unsaturated fats should be used.

Carbohydrates—Complex carbohydrates like starches and dietary fiber should be included.

Sodium—Mild to moderate sodium restriction (1–2g/day) should be done.

Potassium and calcium—Sufficient amounts of foods rich in potassium and calcium should be included in the diet.

Dietary Management

Energy—Increased calorie intake especially in the form of carbohydrate and fat has been shown to significantly increase sympathetic nervous system (SNS) activity. An increased SNS activity can elevate blood pressure. About 20 kcal/kg of ideal body weight are prescribed for a sedentary worker and 25 kcal/kg body weight for moderately active worker. In case of a obese hypertensives, a hypocaloric diet is recommended.

Protein—Intake of 60 g protein daily is necessary to maintain proper nutritional status. Since protein foods are rich in sodium, in severe hypertension a reduction of 20g proteins may be advised as a temporary measure.

Fats—A high intake of animal or hydrogenated fats is usually avoided as these patients are more prone to atherosclerosis or other coronary heart diseases. About 20g vegetable oil is permitted.

Carbohydrates—Easily available complex carbohydrates play an important role in the management of high blood pressure. About 60 to 65 per cent of the energy should come from the carbohydrate foods.

Sodium—Sodium restriction along with weight reduction is effective in controlling mild to moderate hypertension. Increased intake of sodium in diet leads to increased cardiac output thus elevating the blood pressure. Restricted sodium and a decrease in the sodium/potassium ratio in the diet are preferred. Moderate sodium restriction that is 2–3 g/day reduces diastolic pressure 6–10mm Hg and enhances the blood pressure lowering effect of diuretic therapy.

Potassium—Potassium intake should be adequate and potassium rich foods such as fruits and vegetables should be included in the diet. Potassium's role in hypertension is actually important and is the result of complex interplay with sodium. For example, low levels of potassium cause the body to retain sodium and water and this can elevate blood pressure. 3500 mg of potassium is required daily and fruits and vegetables should be taken liberally to meet the potassium requirements.

Foods to be avoided

1. Salt in cooking or at the table.
2. Monosodium glutamate, baking powder, sodium bicarbonate and sodium benzoate.
3. Salt preserved foods like pickles.
4. Highly salted foods such as potato chips, sauces, frozen peas, shell fish, dry fish, biscuits, breads, cakes, pastries.

Atherosclerosis

Atherosclerosis is a disease affecting the arterial blood vessels. It is commonly referred to as a "hardening" of the arteries and is caused by the formation of multiple plaques within the arteries. The term atherosclerosis has been derived from the Greek word "Ethera" meaning, gruel as the lesions formed have a deposit of yellow porridge like material. It is the nodular accumulation of a soft, flaky, yellowish material at the center of large plaques, near the lumen of the artery. It is a pathological process in coronary arteries, cerebral arteries and aorta that are responsible for coronary heart diseases and stroke.

Arteriosclerosis results from a deposition of tough, rigid collagen inside the vessel wall and around the atheroma. This increases the stiffness and decreases the elasticity of the artery wall.

Arteriosclerosis means, degenerative changes in the arteries, characterized by thickening of the vessel walls and accumulation of calcium with consequent loss of elasticity and lessened blood flow.

Atherosclerosis is a common form of arteriosclerosis in which fatty substances form a deposit of plaque on the inner lining of arterial walls.

Arteriolosclerosis (hardening of small arteries, the arterioles) is the result of collagen deposition, but also muscle wall thickening and deposition of protein .

Causes and Risk Factors

- Age
- Sex
- Smoking
- Obesity
- A diet high in fats, sugar or salt
- Stress
- High blood pressure
- High levels of cholesterol
- Kidney disease
- Personal or family history of heart disease

Symptoms

- Chest pain when a coronary artery is involved
- Leg pain when a leg artery is involved
- Atherosclerosis often shows symptoms in a very late stage when the flow within a blood vessel has become seriously compromised.

Prevention and Treatment

- Lowering cholesterol levels
- Lowering blood pressure
- Stop smoking
- Losing weight
- Start exercising Myocardial infarction

Energy—Hypocaloric diet

Fat—Low fat, low cholesterol diet with monounsaturated fatty acids

Proteins— More of vegetable proteins

Carbohydrates—More of complex carbohydrates and water soluble fibre (whole pulses, legumes, beans, oats, fruits and vegetables)

Minerals and vitamins—From fruits and vegetables

Sodium—Low sodium diet

Myocardial Infarction

Myocardial infarction is a disease that occurs when the blood supply to a part of the heart is interrupted, causing death of the heart tissue. The term myocardial infarction is derived from myocardium (the heart muscle) and infarction (tissue death due to oxygen deficiency or ischemia). It is the leading cause of death for both men and women all over the world. In this disease there is severe damage to the heart and it is no longer able to maintain the normal circulation to supply nutrients and oxygen to the tissues or to dispose off carbon-dioxide and other wastes. Prompt medical measures including bed rest, oxygen and blood therapy are essential to relieve the strain to the heart.

Causes and Risk Factors

- High blood pressure
- Too much fat in the diet

- Diabetes
- Smoking
- Obesity
- Age
- Sex
- Heredity

Symptoms

- Fainting
- Nausea or vomiting
- Sweating
- Anxiety
- Chest pain
- Shortness of breath
- Cough
- Dizziness

Prevention and Diet

- Eat a low fat diet rich in fruits and vegetables and low in animal fat
- Lose weight if overweight
- Exercise daily or several times a week by walking and other exercises to improve heart fitness
- Control blood pressure
- Control total cholesterol levels
- Stop smoking

Congestive Heart Failure

Congestive heart failure, also called as congestive cardiac failure, is a condition that results from any structural or functional cardiac disorder that impairs the ability of the heart. It is a condition in which the heart cannot pump out all of the blood that enters it, which leads to an accumulation of blood in the vessels and fluid in the body tissues. In this condition the heart failure is caused by the loss of pumping power of the heart. It results in fluid collection in the body (oedema). Congestive heart failure often develops gradually over several years, although it also can happen suddenly. It can be treated by drugs and in some cases, by surgery. In chronic coronary heart diseases, congestive heart failure may develop over a period of time. The heart muscle myocardium gets progressively weakened and is not able to maintain normal cardiac output and thus normal circulation.

Causes and Risk Factors

- Hypertension (high blood pressure)
- Lung disease
- Overweight
- Smoking cigarettes
- Congenital heart disease

Symptoms

- Weight gain
- Swelling of feet and ankles
- Shortness of breath
- Fatigue, weakness, faintness
- Difficulty in sleeping
- Irregular or rapid pulse
- Cardiac oedema and pulmonary oedema
- Decreased alertness or concentration
- Swelling of the abdomen
- Loss of appetite, indigestion
- Nausea and vomiting

Prevention and Treatment

- One should take the medications as directed.
- Limit salt and sodium intake
- Treat high cholesterol with diet, exercise, and medication if necessary.
- Don't smoke
- Stay active
- Lose weight if overweight
- Get enough rest, including after exercise, eating, or other activities. This allows heart to rest as well. Keep feet elevated to decrease swelling

Energy—Hypocaloric diet

Protein—Normal i.e. 1g/kg body weight

Fat—Low fat, more of MUFA and PUFA

Carbohydrates—Easily digestible carbohydrates

Sodium—Sodium restriction

Fluid—About 1.5–2 lt/day. But in severe oedema the intake is restricted

Dietary Management

In the initial phase of the heart diseases, the basic objective is cardiac rest and a strict dietary management is usually required. Objectives of diet modifications in cardiac disorders are:–

1. To give adequate nourishment with minimum work effort
2. Maximum rest for the heart
3. To prevent further damage to the heart
4. To restore the damaged heart to normal functioning

5. Maintenance of good nutrition
6. Acceptability
7. To relieve strain to the heart
8. To prevent and eliminate edema

To achieve the above objectives the diet is further modified in energy value and texture.

The diet used is basically normal diet, which is low in cholesterol and saturated fat, or the prudent diet. Low calorie, low fat, particularly low saturated fat, low cholesterol, high PUFA, MUFA with omega-6 and omega-3 fatty acids, low carbohydrates, normal protein, minerals, high fiber and vitamins are suggested.

Energy

1. During the initial recovery period, the diet may be limited to about 1200 to 1500 kcal.
2. The total calories should be restricted so as to reduce the weight according to what is expected normal for the height, age and sex.
3. Mild degree of weight loss for the cardiac patient of normal weight is also recommended. Usually a 1000–1200 kcal diet is suitable for an obese patient in bed.
4. For the initial few days 800–1000 kcal/day may be recommended and progress to 1200 kcal/day afterwards while the patient is still at bed rest. Obese or overweight patients experience symptomatic relief after weight reduction.
5. Loss of weight by the obese leads to a considerable reduction in work of the heart because the BMR is at the lower level. There is a slowing of the heart rate. A drop in blood pressure and thereby, improved cardiac efficiency.
6. It is advisable to under nourish the patient for first two days after the heart attack. Ingestion of food involves increased cardiac output so as to meet the metabolic demands for the digestion, absorption and assimilation of foods. Therefore, by giving a hypo

caloric diet or by restricting the food intake the metabolic activity can be decreased to a level that the weakened heart can accommodate without extra strain.

7. In the rehabilitative stage calories are adjusted as necessary to bring about weight change if needed.
8. Those patients whose weight is at desirable levels are permitted a maintenance level of calories during convalescence.

Fat—The fats are restricted to no more then 20 percent of the total calories consumed. Levels as low as 20 percent are tolerated without side effects. It is not desirable to restrict all forms of fat as severe restriction results in mental and physical depression. Since both the amount and type of fat have to be modified, the general diet is suitable for the patient. It should be low in calories, less than 20 percent of energy should be derived from fats.

PUFA—The important polyunsaturated fatty acids are linoleic acid and alpha-linolenic acid. Omega-6 fatty acids, linoleic acid lowers both total cholesterol and LDL cholesterol levels. However a very high level of linoleic acid also lowers HDL cholesterol levels. Omega-3 polyunsaturated fatty acids lower LDL cholesterol and total serum cholesterol levels but not the HDL levels. In vegetarians excessive intake of linoleic acid is avoided. Linoleic acid prevents accumulation of cholesterol in blood serum and in the walls of blood vessels.

The **polyunsaturated** fatty acids (PUFA) promote esterification of cholesterol and convert it into easily utilizable form. PUFA also decrease the production of LDL and VLDL, which are associated with the increased risk of coronary heart diseases. Fish contain a very good amount of PUFA (omega-3). Consumption of 100–200 g of fish two to three times a week helps in preventing heart diseases (NIN, Hyderabad, 1992).

Monounsaturated fatty acids are present in vegetable sources such as olive oil, canola oil, almond oil and groundnut oil. They lower LDL without lowering HDL cholesterol.

Mustard oil and **soybean** oil are rich in omega-3 (alpha-linolenic acid). Safflower oil and corn oil are rich in omega-6 (linoleic acid).

Cholesterol—Cholesterol is manufactured in the liver in the amounts required by the body to perform its various functions. Liver synthesizes as much as 2g of cholesterol/day. Cholesterol level in the diet should not exceed 300mg. If Blood cholesterol levels are above 260 mg/dl it is almost impossible to bring about drop by diet. The advantage of the vegetarian diet is that it is low in calories, fat and cholesterol. It has a high P/S ratio and it has adequate fiber, which helps in binding cholesterol and increases the excretion of cholesterol. Vegetable oils diminish the plasma cholesterol with the help of polyunsaturated fatty acids and plant sterols that inhibits the cholesterol absorption.

Carbohydrates—Carbohydrates should contribute rest of the energy in the diet. Easily digestible carbohydrates should be included so as to reduce the work of the heart to the minimum. Since total calories are restricted, carbohydrate intake might be reduced.

Proteins—Normal intake of protein that is 1g/kg body weight is advised for the maintenance of body tissue protein. Animal proteins are not suggested for atherosclerosis patient. Since total fat, animal fat, organ meats, eggs and seafoods are restricted.

Vitamins and Minerals—Normal allowances of vitamins and minerals are recommended. Vitamin-A deficiency may occur. Therefore, supplement of vitamin-A is essential.

Cardiac Oedema

The fluid imbalance resulting in cardiac oedema is caused by many different mechanisms, which are as follows:

1. The normal capillary fluid shift mechanism is responsible for maintaining the flow of fluids throughout the body. This mechanism fails to operate properly in congestive heart failure. The failing heart is not able to pump out the blood fast resulting in blood accumulation in the vascular system of the right side of the heart thus affecting normal circulation. This affects the normal flow of fluid between the tissues space and blood vessels

Vitamin C

Arteries are the large, elastic blood vessels, which carry blood away from the heart, both to the lungs (deoxygenated blood) and to the rest of the body (oxygenated blood). They are composed of three layers, which, in varying degree are made up of various structural components, the most important of which is collagen—a soft, pliable, elastic substance, which allows the artery to stretch and contract under the control of muscle systems.

Like all other cells in the body, the artery cells are constantly under attack from free radicals and other cell-damaging forces and are in a continual state of replacement and repair. As a consequence, they need a constant supply of new collagen to replace the damaged cells. Collagen is made of a number of components, especially vitamin C.

When there is insufficient vitamin C in the body, new collagen cannot be formed to repair the damaged artery cells. This causes a problem for the body. It, therefore, has to find something else to repair the damage and uses cholesterol. Molecules of cholesterol actually bind to the damaged sites, preventing blood loss and its disastrous consequences. As time goes on, and body does not get enough vitamin C, this process repeats itself (in the absence of Vitamin C) and gradually the arteries become clogged, restricting the blood flow.

and instead of the fluids being returned to the circulation it starts accumulating in the tissue spaces causing oedema.

2. Aldosterone and anti-diuretic hormone that control water balance in the body also leads to the cardiac oedema in congestive heart failure. The aldosterone and anti diuretic hormones are associated with the prevention of the loss of salt and water. Its contribution to the retention of sodium in patients with congestive heart failure, cirrhosis, and the nephrotic syndrome has also been established.

3. Increased free cell calcium, reduced blood circulation depresses the cell metabolism resulting in cell protein breakdown and release of potassium in the cell. Increased amount of intracellular free potassium increases the osmotic pressure. In order to balance this increase as well as to prevent cell dehydration, there is an increase of sodium in the extra cellular fluid and thus excess of fluid eventually leads to water retention.

4. Cardiogenic oedema also results from an increase in capillary hydrostatic pressure (either pulmonary or systemic). This increase produces a reduction in the plasma colloid osmotic pressure-capillary pressure gradient, facilitating the accumulation of fluid in the interstitial spaces and reducing the circulating plasmatic volume.

Treatment

The aim of treatment in cardiac oedema is to secure maximum rest for the heart and to remove oedema. Basis of treatment are:–

1. Complete rest.
2. Administration of diuretics.
3. Diet prescription, low in sodium and energy.

Sodium—The diet has to be restricted in sodium because of cardiac oedema. A mild sodium restriction of 2–3 g/day is recommended.

Low sodium diet consisting of 2 g is usually prescribed. As in many cardiac disorders there are chances of water retention. When sodium is restricted, other sources of iodine should be prescribed. A severe restriction of iodine also reduces the intake of vitamin-A because egg and green leafy vegetables are high in sodium, are restricted. In severe oedema the intake of fluid is also restricted.

Sodium restricted diets have been divided into the following:

a) Mild Sodium Restriction (2 to 3 g)

Salt may be used lightly in cooking, assuming that fresh foods are used, but no added salt and salty processed foods are allowed.

b) Moderate Sodium Restriction (1000 mg)

No salt is used in cooking, and no added salt or salty foods are used. Beginning at this level, some control of foods with natural sodium is started. Foods higher in sodium are limited. Fresh foods are used rather than those processed with salt. Salt free baked products can be used. Foods with higher sodium content are only used in moderate portions.

c) Strict Sodium Restriction (500 mg)

The natural sodium food sources of meat, milk and egg are used in small portions. Milk is limited to two cups in any form. Vegetables containing higher sodium are not allowed.

Diet and Feeding Pattern—As there is congestion of digestive organs, each feed should be small in quantity and easy to digest. To provide adequate nutrition, number of feeds should be increased. The general principals of diet and feeding are the same almost as in the case of all the heart diseases. Fixed meal timings with adequate rest after meals is important. Foods rich in fats, saturated fats and cholesterol should be avoided. Natural foods should not be restricted.

Duration of Meal and Exercise—3–4 small meals are suggested instead of two big meals. The evening meals should be consumed two hours before going to the bed. Regular exercise and relaxed mental attitude helps to reduce pressure. Smoking and drinking alcohol should be stopped.

Sodium content of foods per 100gm

Less than 25 mg	25–50mg	50–100mg	More than 100mg
Amla, bitter gourd, bottle gourd, brinjal, cabbage, colocasia, cow pea, cucumber, French beans, grapes, guava, honey, horse gram, lady fingers, maida, milk (buffalo), oil, onion, orange, papaya, peas, plantain, potato, pumpkin, ragi, sapota, semolina, sugar, sweet potato tomato (ripe), vermicelli, wheat, yam.	Apple, banana, Bengal gram (whole), black gram dal, broad beans, carrots, cream, green gram dal, lentil (whole), mango (green), mango (ripe), mutton, raisins, red gram dal, tomato (green).	Water melon, beetroot, beef, Bengal gram dal, cauliflower, chicken, coriander leaves, fenugreek, field beans, lettuce, liver, prawns, red gram (tender).	Amaranth, bacon, egg, knoll khol, lobster, spinach.

Easy to Learn

- Eat a healthy diet with lots of fruits, vegetables, whole grains, and a limited amount of red meats. Get at least 5 (more is even better) servings of fruits and vegetables a day.

- Make fruits and vegetables part of every meal. Frozen or canned can be used when fresh isn't available.
- Eat vegetables as snacks.
- Cut down "bad" fats (trans-fatty acids and saturated fats) and consume "good" fats (polyunsaturated and monounsaturated fats like olive oil and canola oil). Cook with oils that contain a lot of polyunsaturated and monounsaturated fats, such as olive or canola oil.
- Choose chicken, fish, or beans instead of red meat and cheese.
- Choose margarines that do not have partially hydrogenated oils. Soft margarines (especially squeeze margarines) have less trans-fatty acids than stick margarines.
- Eat fewer baked goods that are store-made and contain partially hydrogenated fats.
- Take a daily multivitamin containing 400 micrograms of folate. Folate is good for heart.
- Eat breakfast cereal that is fortified with folate. Check the label to be sure.
- Eat fruits and vegetables that are rich in folate, such as oranges, orange juice, and green leafy vegetables.
- Choose non-alcoholic beverages, like juices and sodas at meals and parties.
- Avoid occasions centered around alcohol.
- Avoid making alcohol an essential part of family gatherings.
- Constipation should always be avoided and can be relieved through judicious use of fruits and vegetables. The choice of food must be restricted to those, which are non-distending. There is variation in individual's tolerance in this regard.
- Eggs can be included in the diet in restricted amounts. It is also safe to include shrimps and crabs to a low cholesterol diet. Skimmed milk can be given as it has cholesterol-lowering effect.

- Small, soft, frequent feedings and moderate food restriction per meal would also prevent distention of the stomach. During this stage the patient must not even be permitted to feed himself. When the patient's condition improves, he may be given foods, which are easy to chew and digest.
- All liquids are served at room temperature. Beverages containing caffeine are omitted because of their stimulating effect on heart rate.

Review Questions

1. What do you mean by cardiovascular diseases?
2. What is myocardial infarction? Write down its symptoms and dietary management.
3. What are LDL and HDL? Differentiate between the two.
4. How can we cure hypertension?
5. Write down the various risk factors, which can cause heart problems.

Liver and its Disorders

Introduction

Liver is body's chemical workshop. The adult human liver normally weighs between 1.3–2.0 kg, and it is a soft, pinkish-brown "boomerang shaped" organ. It is the second largest organ (the largest organ being the skin) and the largest gland within the human body. It is located in the right side of the body under the lower ribs and is divided into four lobes of unequal size. Two large vessels carry blood to the liver. The hepatic artery comes from the heart and carries blood rich in oxygen. The portal vein brings the liver blood rich in nutrients absorbed from the small intestine. These vessels divide into capillaries. These capillaries reach the thousands of lobules of the liver. Each lobule is composed of hepatocytes, and as blood passes through, they are able to monitor, add, and remove substances from it. The blood then leaves the liver via the hepatic

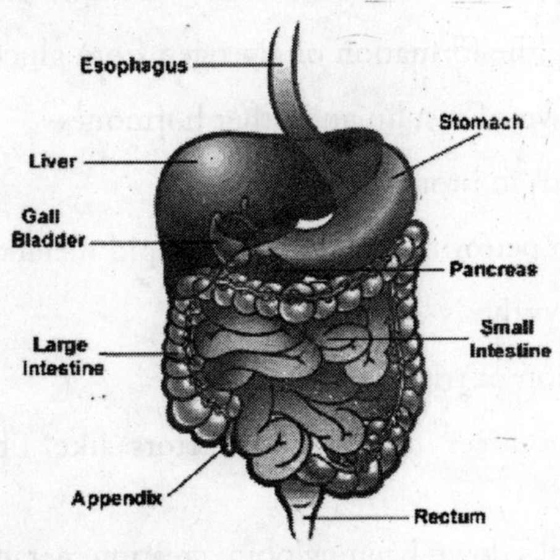

vein, returns to the heart, and is ready to be pumped to the rest of the body.

The liver makes a kind of bed for the gallbladder (which stores bile). It is a multifunctional organ, which plays an important role in carbohydrates, fat and protein metabolism.

Functions of the Liver

The body depends on the liver to perform a number of vital functions and they can be divided into three basic categories i.e. **regulation**, **synthesis**, and **secretion** of many substances important in maintaining the body's normal state, storage of important nutrients, and purification, transformation, and clearance of waste products, drugs, and toxins. The various functions of the liver are given below :

- The liver produces and excretes bile required for emulsifying fats. Some of the bile drains directly into the duodenum, and some is stored in the gallbladder.
- The liver performs several roles in carbohydrate metabolism:
- Gluconeogenesis (the synthesis of glucose from non carbohydrate sources like amino acids, lactate or glycerol)
- Glycogenolysis (the breakdown of glycogen into glucose)
- Glycogenesis (the formation of glycogen from glucose)
- The breakdown of insulin and other hormones
- The liver helps in protein metabolism.
- The liver also performs several roles in lipid metabolism:
- Cholesterol synthesis
- The production of triglycerides (fats)
- The liver produces coagulation factors like fibrinogen and prothrombin
- The liver breaks down haemoglobin, creating metabolites that are added to bile as pigment (bilirubin and biliverdin).

- The liver breaks down toxic substances and most medicinal products in a process called drug metabolism. This sometimes results in toxication, when the metabolite is more toxic than its precursor.
- The liver converts ammonia to urea.
- The liver stores minerals and vitamins like vitamin b12, iron and copper
- The liver is responsible for immunological effects—the reticuloendothelial system of the liver contains many immunologically active cells, which act as a 'sieve' for antigens carried to it via the portal system.

The liver is designed to store important substances such as glucose in the form of glycogen. The liver also stores fat-soluble vitamins (vitamins A, D, E and K), folate, vitamin B_{12}, and minerals such as copper and iron. However, excessive accumulation of certain substances can be harmful. For example, patients with an inherited condition known as Wilson's disease cannot secrete copper into bile normally and usually have a low blood level of the copper-binding protein ceruloplasmin. Retained copper accumulates in the liver and can lead to cirrhosis.

Agents responsible for Liver Damage

(1) **Dietary Deficiency**—Fatty changes seen in the liver may be attributed to a low protein intake. Children suffering from kwashiorkor also suffer from such changes. Fatty changes in liver are common whenever there is a high proportion of fat in metabolic mixtures as in uncontrolled diabetes, starvation, in some cases of obesity and when too much carbohydrate has been infused during intravenous feeding. These changes are easily reversible and not followed by fibrosis.

(2) **Infective Agents**—Infective agents like viruses have been found to cause liver disorders. Viruses can cause infection and damage the

liver. Hepatitis A virus is excreted in the stools of patients or carriers of the disease and spread through oral faecal route. Poor personal hygiene can also cause this infection.

Hepatitis B virus causes homologous serum jaundice. It arises after transfusion of blood or blood products obtained from a donor, who is a carrier of the disease. Improper sterilized needles can also cause hepatitis B, thus, is common among drug addicts.

(3) **Toxic Agents**—Toxins such as alcohol, drugs, or poisons can cause liver disorders directly by damaging liver tissue or indirectly by reducing defenses or stimulating an autoimmune response.

Alcohol—Alcohol is primarily metabolized by the liver, and these metabolites can cause liver damage. The risk of hepatic toxicity increases if more than 40 grams, or about four drinks, are consumed per day. Alcohol is also known to have direct action on lipid metabolism in the liver by enhancing fatty acid synthesis, decreasing fatty acid oxidation, and producing specific stimulation to triglyceride formation.

Drug—Numerous medications can damage the liver, ranging from mild, asymptomatic alteration in liver to hepatic failure and death. Liver toxicity may or may not be dose-related. Paracetamole, dilantin (an anti-convulsant) and isoniazid (an anti-tuberculosis agent) are examples of drugs that can cause liver disorders.

Chemicals/Poisons—Both environmental and industrial toxins can cause a wide variety of changes in the liver. Workers in chemical factories are at more risk to liver damage because of more exposure to chemicals.

(4) **Metabolic Disorders**—Problems with metabolic processes in the liver can be either congenital (present at birth) or acquired. Some of these disorders, such as Wilson's disease and haemochromatosis, can be present as hepatitis or cirrhosis and must be distinguished from other causes of these forms of liver disease.

Wilson's disease is a rare inherited condition, mostly affecting young people that are characterized by an inability to excrete copper into bile, resulting in the toxic accumulation of copper in the liver and nervous system. Manifestations include liver disease and neuropsychiatric symptoms.

Haemochromatosis is an iron overload syndrome causing iron deposits and consequent damage to various organs, including the liver (cirrhosis), heart (heart failure), pancreas (diabetes), and pituitary gland (decreased sex drive and impotence). The disease may be due to an inherited increase in gut absorption of iron or to multiple blood transfusions, since iron is normally found in circulating red blood cells.

Jaundice

Jaundice is not a disease but rather a sign that can occur in many different diseases. Jaundice is the yellowish staining of the skin and sclerae (the whites of the eyes) that is caused by high levels of bilirubin. The colour of the skin and sclerae vary depending on the level of bilirubin. When the bilirubin level is mildly elevated, they are yellowish. When the bilirubin level is high, they tend to be brown. Damage to liver cells leads to increase in billirubin resulting in jaundice. Normal plasma billirubin levels are 2–8 mg / litre of blood (serum bilirubin 0.1–0.25 mg/100ml).

After 120 days of life cycle, RBCs (red blood cells) are broken down through a complex chemical reaction and billirubin is produced. This is excreted in stools and urine along with bile. Problems like increased destruction of RBCs, decreased functioning of liver or obstruction to flow of bile from the liver can result in jaundice.

R.B.C's → Haem+globin → Bilirubin+iron → Excreted in the faeces and urine

Mild rises in bilirubin may be caused by

- Hemolysis or increased breakdown of red blood cells.
- Gilbert's syndrome—a genetic disorder of bilirubin metabolism which can result in mild jaundice, found in about 5 percent of the population.

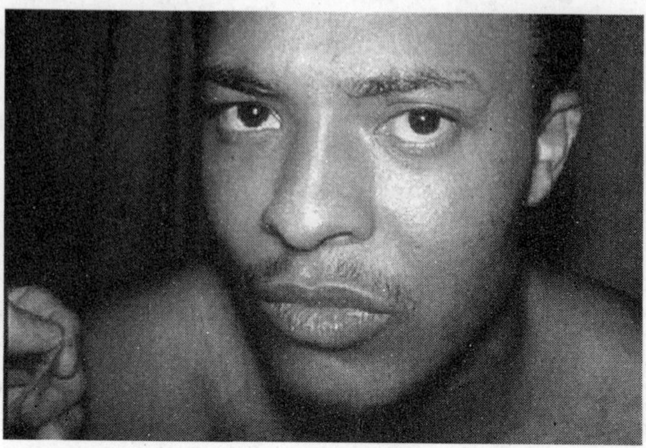

A jaundice patient

Types of Jaundice

(1) **Hepatocellular** jaundice is due to damage to the hepatic cells by toxins or infective agents interfering with the uptake and conjugation of billirubin by the cells or because of the blockage of the bile canaliculi.

(2) **Prehepatic (Haemolytic)** jaundice is due to increased billirubin levels in the blood because of excessive destruction of red blood cells. This is more common in new borns i.e. neonatal jaundice. It may also arise from congenital defects like thalessaemia, sickle cell anaemia, incompatible blood transfusions or intake of certain drugs.

(3) **Post hepatic (Obstructive)** jaundice is due to an obstruction in bile flow between the liver and duodenum. It is mostly common in case of patient suffering from gallstones or cancer of liver or pancreas.

Other symptoms of liver disorders include lassitude, weakness, fatigue, fever, anorexia, weight loss, abdominal pain, flatulence, nausea, vomiting etc.

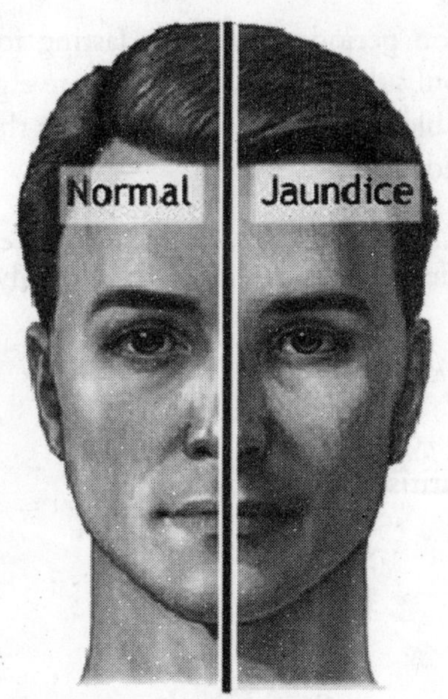

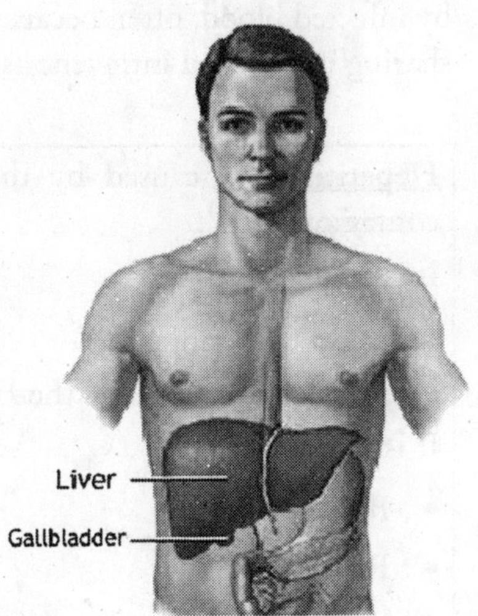

Hepatitis

Hepatitis is a gastroenterological disease. It is an infectious disease characterised by inflammation and degeneration of liver cells. Hepatitis is mainly of two types i.e. viral induced and drug induced. Viral hepatitis is more common and may be either infective (Type A) or serum hepatitis (Type B). The hepatitis A is mild and easily progresses to chronic stage where as Type B, can lead to serious hepatic damage.

Infective Hepatitis

The main transmission of hepatitis A virus is through contaminated food or water and is sometimes found in areas of poor sanitation and inadequate housing. It is only infectious during the incubation period and is not transmitted by carriers. It can also be transmitted through infected blood products.

Serum Hepatitis

Hepatitis B has a longer incubation period, sometimes lasting for several months. It is transmitted only through parenteral route e.g. by infected blood, often because of blood transfusions or through the sharing of infected intravenous needles.

Hepatitis A is caused by the Hepatitis A Virus and is highly contagious.

It is transmitted by:

- faecal-oral contact

Hepatitis B is caused by the Hepatitis B Virus [HBV].

It is found in:

- Blood
- Faecal matter
- Saliva
- Urine

Symptoms

Hepatitis is an inflammation of the liver characterized by malaise, joint aches, abdominal pain, vomiting 2–3 times per day for the first 5 days, defecation, loss of appetite, dark urine, fever, enlarged liver and jaundice. The pre-jaundice stage is Preicteric stage and is the period when non-specific symptoms are seen but this is not manifested clinically. Even during this phase virus is excreted in faeces and is capable of infecting others. This is followed by Icteric stage when symptoms like jaundice are seen. In children, symptoms like jaundice are not commonly seen and only a biochemical test can confirm the occurrence of hepatitis. This is known as anicteric form of jaundice. Generally, symptoms may subside after 2–8 weeks, though a complete recovery may take longer. If the liver is damaged the severity and duration of disease is increased.

Different forms of Hepatitis

Mild hepatitis	Moderate hepatitis	Acute hepatitis	Chronic hepatitis
Usually no jaundice is seen in such cases and all characteristic symptoms of infective hepatitis may not be present. Only biochemical tests confirm the disease but there is a slight increase in conjugated serum billirubin levels.	It is also known as acute icteric form, this is the most common form where the preicteric and icteric stages are seen. All characteristic symptoms and biochemical changes are observed. The patient recovers completely with proper treatment.	In acute hepatitis there is acute necrosis of liver cells, such a condition is very rare and can prove fatal.	If timely treatment is not given, the above-mentioned types of hepatitis may develop into chronic hepatitis. Progressive damage to cells may occur leading to cirrhosis of liver.

Dietary Modifications

The basis of treatment is adequate rest and requires dietary modifications. The objectives of diet therapy are to relieve symptoms, to aid in regeneration of liver cells and to prevent further liver damage.

To achieve the above objectives the following dietary modifications are made:

Energy

Since, the patient initially may not be able to eat such large quantities of food due to illness and only 1500–2000 kcal will be acceptable. Gradually energy intake will be increased 20–30 percent more than normal intake. Since the patient is advised bed rest. His actual daily expenditure is reduced and therefore the recommended intake of energy under normal condition will be sufficient to meet extra needs. A high energy is needed to promote weight gain and to ensure maximum protein utilization.

Protein

It is important to have a protein of high biological value to insure the maximum utilization of protein, preferably supplemented with protein of vegetable origin. In mild to moderate cases, a high intake of 1.5–2g/kg of body weight is suggested. On the other hand in acute cases with excessive liver damage the protein intake may have to be decreased even below normal. Protein intake needs to overcome a negative nitrogen balance to promote regeneration of liver cells and to prevent fatty infiltration of liver. However the damaged liver may not be able to tolerate a high protein load because the conversion of ammonia to urea gets affected and thus there are chances of hepatic coma. Therefore, the protein intake depends on extent of liver damage.

Carbohydrates

A high carbohydrate diet is recommended to provide more of energy, to build up glycogen stores in liver as protection against fatty infiltration and for their protein sparing action. So a daily intake of 300 to 400 g of carbohydrates of simple nature should be given.

Fats

In liver disorder, digestion of fat is affected because of impaired bile action. In mild to moderate cases 35 to 45 g total fat/day may be given. In severe cases accompanied by liver damage total fat may be restricted to 20 to 30 g/day. More than the quantity the quality of fat should be modified. Emulsified fats such as milk fat should be given. Medium chain triglycerides present in coconut are also better tolerated.

Minerals and Vitamins

A judicious intake of minerals and vitamins should be there. Diet should provide all minerals particularly calcium and iron in adequate amount because of the increased tissue catabolism. The availability of fat-soluble vitamins is low because of decreased intake and impaired absorption of fat. Therefore, care should be taken to include carotene rich foods like green leafy vegetables, deep yellow, orange fruits and vegetables in the diet.

Foods to be included	Foods to be restricted
Sugar, glucose, honey, cereals, pulses milk and milk products, egg, fruits and vegetables excluding strongly flavoured foods.	Fats, oils, nuts, oil seeds, strongly flavoured vegetables and meat apart from these foods, intake of alcohol during the attack.

Except the mode of transmission of virus, hepatitis A and B are very similar

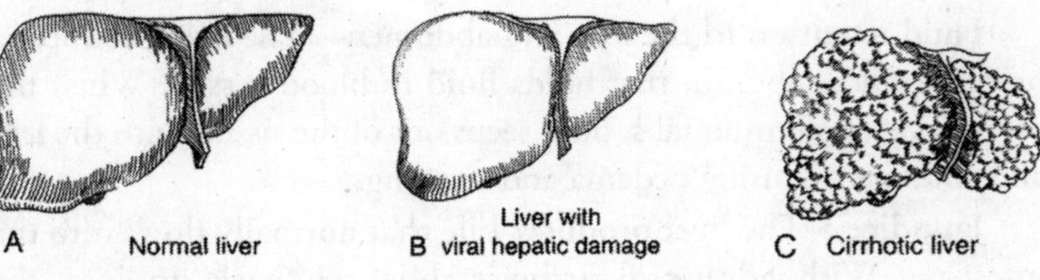

Source: Kathleen M.L., Page-64

Cirrhosis is a condition that causes irreversible scarring of the liver and is a consequence of chronic liver disease. It is a disease of the liver in which fibrous connective tissue replaces the functioning hepatic cells. It is characterised by destruction of liver cells, distortion of normal lobules with growth of fibrous tissue and nodular regeneration of cells, following fatty degeneration. Cirrhosis is the most serious of all the liver diseases.

The scar tissue that forms in cirrhosis harms the liver and blocks the flow of blood through the organ. The loss of normal liver tissue slows the processing of nutrients, hormones, drugs, and toxins by the liver.

Cirrhosis may be of three types

(1) **Laennec's Cirrhosis**–chronic alcoholics are more prone to this type of cirrhosis.

(2) **Post-necrotic Scarring,** is observed in few cases of acute infective hepatitis who do not respond to treatment.

(3) **Biliary Cirrhosis**, which occurs due to obstruction in the bile duct. Once dense vascular and fibrosis bands have formed, scarring becomes permanent.

Symptoms

Many people with cirrhosis have no symptoms in the early stages of the disease. However, as scar tissue replaces healthy cells, liver function starts to fail and a person may experience the following symptoms:

Fluid retention in the legs and abdomen—The liver produces a protein, called albumin that holds fluid in blood vessels. When the blood level of albumin falls, fluid seeps out of the tissues into the legs and abdomen, causing oedema and swelling.

Jaundice—The liver produces bile that normally flows into the intestine. With advanced cirrhosis, bile can back up into the blood, causing the skin and eyes to turn yellow and the urine to darken.

Itching—Certain types of cirrhosis, such as chronic bile duct blockage, can cause itching.

Gallstones—Cirrhosis causes the abnormal metabolism of bile pigment. Because of this, gallstones develop twice as often in cirrhosis patients as in those without the disorder.

Coagulation Defects—The liver makes certain proteins that help clot blood. When these proteins are deficient, excessive or prolonged bleeding happens.

Mental Function Change—The liver processes toxins from the intestine. When these substances escape into the bloodstream, as occurs in severe cases of cirrhosis, a variety of changes in mental function can develop.

As the disease progresses, complications may develop. In some people, these may be the first signs of the disease.

Causes

Cirrhosis can be caused by many things. It can result from direct injury to the liver cells (i.e., hepatitis) or from indirect injury via inflammation or obstruction to bile ducts. Common causes of cirrhosis are as follows:

Alcohol—Using alcohol in excess is the most common cause of cirrhosis. There is an association between liver disease and chronic alcoholism and malnutrition. Chronic alcoholics, have a long stranding inadequate food intake leading to malnutrition and necrosis of liver cells and subsequently cirrhosis.

Chronic Viral Hepatitis—Type B and Type C hepatitis, and perhaps other viruses, can infect and damage the liver over a prolonged time and eventually cause cirrhosis.

Chronic Bile Duct Blockage—This condition can occur at birth or develop later in life. When the bile ducts outside the liver become narrowed and blocked, can lead to cirrhosis.

Wilson's Disease or Haemochromatosis—Abnormal Storage of Copper (Wilson's Disease) or Iron (Haemochromatosis) can also lead to cirrhosis. These metals are present in all body cells. When abnormal amounts of them accumulate in the liver, scarring and cirrhosis may develop.

Drugs and Toxins—Prolonged exposure to certain chemicals or drugs can scar the liver.

Autoimmune Hepatitis—This chronic inflammation occurs when the body's protective antibodies fail to recognize the liver as its own tissue. The antibodies injure the liver cells as though they were a foreign protein or bacteria.

Diagnosis

The doctor often can diagnose cirrhosis from the patient's symptoms and from laboratory tests like blood test. The purpose of these tests is to find out if liver disease is present. In some cases, other tests that take pictures of the liver are performed such as the computerized axial tomography (CAT) scan, ultrasound, and the radioisotope liver/spleen scan. Biopsy can also be done. Sometimes cirrhosis is diagnosed during surgery when the doctor is able to see the entire liver. The liver also can be inspected through a laparoscope, a viewing device that is inserted through a tiny incision in the abdomen.

Treatment

Treatment of cirrhosis is aimed to stop the development of scar tissue in the liver and prevent complications. When cirrhosis is due to an identifiable cause, treatment programs may be specific, such as for management of hepatitis B and C, or steroids and immunosuppressive agents for auto-immune chronic active hepatitis.

The cirrhotic patient is at increased risk of other infections that may be more severe than the others. Immunizations for hepatitis A, B, influenza, and pneumococcal pneumonia are available and should be administered. Raw seafood may contain bacteria that can cause life-threatening infections and therefore should be avoided.

Complications with treatment

The abnormal accumulation of fluid may cause swelling of the ankles (oedema) and abdomen (ascites). Therefore, patients should reduce the amount of fluid and salt in their diet. Occasionally, the ascites may become infected leading to spontaneous bacterial peritonitis, and require treatment with antibiotics.

When the liver does not efficiently function to cleanse the body of toxins and drugs, the mental state of patients may change dramatically and lead to coma, called **Hepatic Encephalopathy**. Treatment is directed at reducing the protein in the diet, avoiding sedatives and pain medications, and using laxatives and/or antibiotics to decrease the absorption of toxins from the intestines. Sometimes, bleeding from the oesophagus or stomach caused by abnormal veins (varices) may occur and is a life-threatening emergency requiring hospitalization. When complications develop, it may be possible to manage them. When it is likely that liver failure will develop, some patients with cirrhosis are able to undergo liver transplantation.

Dietary Modification

The objectives of dietary modifications are:

(1) To promote regeneration of liver cells

(2) To correct fluid and electrolyte balance

(3) To ractify the nutritional deficiencies

Energy

During the disease the patient becomes malnourished, so the energy requirements are increased. The energy is also required to promote regeneration of liver cells. The actual energy expenditure is reduced as the patient is on bed rest. Therefore, the normal recommended energy intakes are enough to meet the bodily needs.

Protein

About 1.0 to 1.5 g protein per kilogram of body weight is suggested in the absence of hepatic coma (coma that can occur in severe cases of liver diseases). However, if signs of impending coma appear, the protein intake is decreased to 0.3 to 0.5g/kg of body weight, depending on the individual tolerance.These intakes help to overcome malnutrition, regenerating liver cells and replenish plasma proteins. More of the vegetable proteins should be included in the diet as the animal proteins contain more of aromatic amino acids and their catabolism causes more ammonia production, and the damaged hepatic cells may not be able to efficiently convert all the ammonia into urea and because of this reason large amounts of animal proteins in the diet of the patient may lead to **hepatic encephalopathy**.

Hepatic encephalopathy is a complex, potentially reversible neuropsychiatric condition that occurs as a consequence of acute or chronic liver disease. It is characterized by changes in personality, consciousness, behaviour and neuromuscular function.

Carbohydrates

A daily intake of 300 g of carbohydrates mainly in the form of simple carbohydrates like glucose, sugar, fruits and fruit juices, starches like cereals and root vegetables are advised. Foods containing irritating fibres should be eliminated due to presence of oesophageal varices. Thus, dehusked pulses, refined cereals and a low fibre vegetables and fruits should be selected.

Oesophageal varices are "varicose" or swollen veins in the walls of the oesophagus.

Fats

As there is impaired bile secretion in liver diseases, many cirrhotic patients may suffer from malabsorption of fat. A restriction in the fat intake should be suggested for such patients. Moderate amount of fat can be included in the diet to increase the palatability and promote recovery. Emulsified fats and fat containing medium chain triglycerides are better tolerated. The amount of fat to be included in the diet will vary according to the individual's tolerance.

Vitamins

The availability of fat soluble vitamins like vitamin A, D, E and K, is affected due to the decreased intake and impaired absorption of fat.Thus,the diet should include β-carotene rich foods. Supplements of B-group vitamins may have to be provided to replenish liver stores and repair tissue damage.

Minerals

Serum calcium and magnesium levels are lowered in cirrhotic patients and therefore adequate amounts of these minerals should be provided in the diet.

Sodium

Sodium is restricted because of the presence of ascites and oedema. In severe cases, a 500 mg sodium diet is recommended and as the patient recovers, the restriction may be further relaxed. One should be very cautious about cooking salt, baking powder and preserved food products. In case of a patient on diuretic therapy, a liberal sodium intake may be advised.

Gall Bladder Disease

Gallstones are the solid stones formed in the gall bladder from cholesterol, bile salts and calcium. They vary in size from a few millimetres to a few centimetres. Bile is made in the liver, then stored in the gallbladder until the body needs to digest fat. At that time, the gallbladder contracts and pushes the bile into the common bile duct that carries it to the small intestine, where it helps in digestion. Bile contains water, cholesterol, fats, bile salts, proteins, and bilirubin. Bile salts break up fat, and bilirubin gives bile and stool a yellowish colour. If the liquid bile contains too much cholesterol, bile salts, or bilirubin, under certain conditions it hardens into stones. The formation of gallstones is also known as cholelithiasis.

There are three types of Gallstones

Cholesterol stones: Cholesterol stones are formed when bile contains too much cholesterol, too much bilirubin, not enough bile salts, or when the gallbladder does not empty, as it should for some other reason. 95 percent of all gallstones are cholesterol stones. Cholesterol stones are usually yellow-green in colour.

Bilirubin stones are formed from cholesterol and bilirubin.

Pigment stones: The cause of pigment stones is uncertain. They tend to develop in people who have cirrhosis, biliary tract infections, and hereditary blood disorders such as sickle cell anaemia.

Symptoms of Gallstones

Symptoms of gallstones include pain in the stomach or just under the ribs. Often, the pain can make it difficult to breathe or get comfortable. The pain sometimes occurs after a meal, can last for several hours, and can even wake a person from sleep.

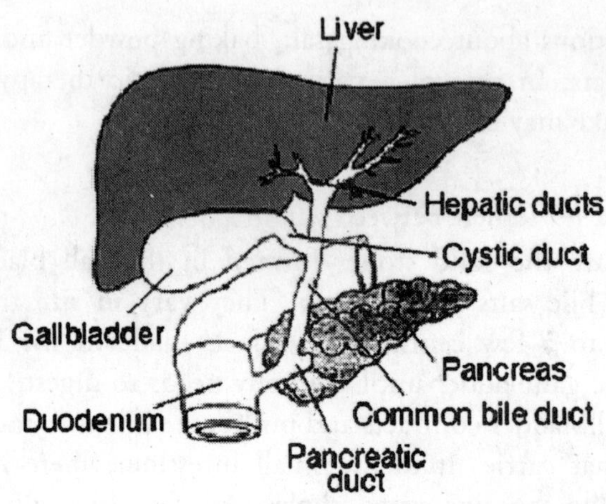

When a stone blocks the duct that drains the gallbladder, other symptoms can include nausea, vomiting, and fever, in addition to pain. Occasionally, gallstones can cause another condition, pancreatitis (inflammation of the pancreas), which blocks the flow of digestive enzymes produced by the pancreas and has similar symptoms like severe pain, loss of appetite, fever, nausea, and vomiting.

The gallbladder and the ducts that carry bile and other digestive enzymes from the liver, gallbladder, and pancreas to the small intestine are called the biliary system.

Factors responsible for Gallstones

It is believed that the mere presence of gallstones may cause more gallstones to develop. However, other factors that contribute to gallstones have been identified, especially for cholesterol stones.

- **Obesity**—Obesity is a major risk factor for gallstones, especially in women. A large clinical study showed that being even moderately overweight increases the risk for developing gallstones. The most likely reason is that obesity tends to reduce the amount of bile salts in bile, resulting in more cholesterol. Obesity also decreases gallbladder emptying.

- **Estrogen**—Excess estrogen during pregnancy, hormone replacement therapy, or birth control pills appear to increase cholesterol levels in bile and decrease gallbladder movement, both of which can lead to gallstones.
- **Gender**—Women between 20 and 60 years of age are twice as likely to develop gallstones as men.
- **Age**—People over age 60 are more likely to develop gallstones than younger people.
- **Cholesterol-lowering drugs**—Drugs that lower cholesterol levels in blood actually increase the amount of cholesterol secreted in bile. This in turn increases the risk of gallstones.
- **Diabetes**—People with diabetes generally have high levels of triglycerides and these in turn increase the risk of gallstones.
- **Rapid weight loss**—As the body metabolizes fat during rapid weight loss, it causes the liver to secrete extra cholesterol into bile, which can cause gallstones.
- **Fasting**—Fasting decreases gallbladder movement, causing the bile to become over concentrated with cholesterol, which can lead to gallstones.

Cholecystitis

Cholecystitis refers to a painful inflammation of the gallbladder's wall.

Causes and Symptoms

In about 95 percent of all cases of cholecystitis, the gallbladder contains gallstones. When these stones block the duct leaving the gallbladder, bile accumulates within the gallbladder. The gallbladder continues to contract, but the bile cannot pass out of the gallbladder in the normal way. Backpressure on the gallbladder, chemical changes from the stagnating bile trapped within the gallbladder, and occasionally bacterial infection, result in damage to the gallbladder wall. As the gallbladder becomes swollen, some areas of the wall do not receive adequate blood flow, and lack of oxygen causes cells to die.

Not all individuals with gallstones will go on to have cholecystitis, since many people never have any symptoms from their gallstones and never know they exist. However, the vast majority of people with cholecystitis will be found to have gallstones. Rare causes of cholecystitis include severe burns or injury, massive systemic infection, severe illness, diabetes, obstruction by a tumor of the duct leaving the gallbladder, and certain uncommon infections of the gallbladder (including bacteria and worms).

Although there are rare reports of patients with chronic cholecystitis who never experience any pain, nearly 100 percent of the time cholecystitis will be diagnosed after a patient has experienced a bout of severe pain in the region of the gallbladder and liver. The pain may be crampy and episodic, or it may be constant. The pain is often described as pushing through to the right upper back and shoulder. Because deep breathing increases the pain, breathing becomes shallow. Fever is often present, and nausea and vomiting are nearly universal.

Diagnosis

Diagnosis of cholecystitis involves a careful abdominal examination. The enlarged, tender gallbladder may be felt through the abdominal wall. Pressure in the upper right corner of the abdomen may cause the patient to stop breathing in, due to an increase in pain. This is called Murphy's sign. Physical examination may also reveal an increased heart rate and an increased rate of breathing.

Blood tests will show an increase in the white blood count, as well as an increase in bilirubin. Ultrasound is used to look for gallstones and to measure the thickness of the gallbladder wall (a marker of inflammation and scarring). A scan of the liver and gallbladder, with careful attention to the system of ducts throughout (called the biliary tree) is also used to find out any obstruction of ducts.

Severe complications of Cholecystitis include:

- Massive infection of the gallbladder, in which the gallbladder becomes filled with pus.

- Perforation of the gallbladder, in which the build-up of material within the gallbladder becomes so great that the wall of the organ bursts, with a resulting abdominal infection called peritonitis.
- Formation of abnormal connections between the gallbladder and other organs (the duodenum, large intestine, stomach), called fistulas.
- Obstruction of the intestine by a very large gallstone.
- Emphysema of the gallbladder, in which certain bacteria that produce gas infect the gallbladder, resulting in stretching of the gallbladder and disruption of its wall by gas

Treatment

Initial treatment of cholecystitis usually requires hospitalization. The patient is given fluids, salts, and sugars through a needle placed in a vein (intravenous or IV). No food or drink is given by mouth, and often a tube, called a nasogastric tube, will need to be passed through the nose and down into the stomach to drain out the excess fluids. If infection is suspected, antibiotics are given.

Ultimately, treatment almost always involves removal of the gallbladder, a surgery called cholecystectomy. This is not usually recommended while the patient is acutely ill, patients with complications usually do require emergency surgery because the death rate increases in these cases. Similarly, those patients who have cholecystitis with no gallstones have about a 50 percent chance of death if the gallbladder is not quickly removed. Most patients, however, do best if surgery is performed after they have been stabilized with fluids, an nasogastric tube, and antibiotics as necessary. When this is possible, gallbladder removal is done within five to six days of diagnosis. In patients who have other serious medical problems that may increase the risks of gallbladder removal surgery, the cholecystectomy is not suggested. In this case, the operation may involve removing obstructing gallstones and draining infected bile, called cholecystotomy.

Prevention

Prevention of cholecystitis is probably best attempted by maintaining a reasonably ideal weight and a good diet.

Dietary Management of Cholecystitis and Cholelithiasis

Usually a low fat, high carbohydrate and moderate protein diet is given. Large meals should be avoided and plenty of fluids should be taken early in the morning, late at night and in between the meals. Since gall bladder is the main organ for metabolization of fat, therefore the main objectives, of the nutritional therapy are—

- To relieve the discomfort of the gall bladder.
- To keep gall bladder at rest by minimizing the contractions.

To achieve the above objectives, following modifications in the diet are made:

Carbohydrate—Since fat is restricted in the diet, carbohydrate sources like, cereals, starches, simple sugars, pulses, fruits etc, should be incorporated, to fulfil the energy requirements.

Protein—Protein intake is kept normal, preferably from vegetarian sources as they contain lesser fat than proteins of animal origin.

Fat—Fat should be restricted in the diet to about 10 to 20 grams. Since fat causes the contractions of the gall bladder and the consequent pain.

Vitamins—Absorption of all fat soluble vitamins that is, A, D, E and K is reduced, so their intake should be increased.

LIST OF FOODS	
FOODS RECOMMENDED	**FOODS TO BE AVOIDED**
Skimmed milk and products	Fatty, fried foods like cutlets, puris, paranthas, pakoras etc.
Beverages like tea, coffee, fruit juices etc	Butter, ghee, cheese, margarine etc.
Cereals like wheat, rice and pulses	Red meats like mutton, ham, sausages, fatty fish
Fruits, Egg white, poultry, sea foods etc.	Cream soups, whole milk and products Fatty desserts like cakes, pastries, ice creams.
Vegetables as tolerated	Chocolates, nuts, dry fruits etc.

Liver damage or obstruction of a bile duct (e.g., gallstone) can lead to cholestasis, (the blockage of bile flow, which causes the malabsorption of dietary fats), steatorrhea (foul-smelling diarrhea caused by non-absorbed fats), and jaundice.

Review Questions

1. "Liver is body's chemical workshop" justify.
2. What is the rationale for treatment of hepatitis A and B?
3. Discuss the dietary management of cirrhosis.
4. Write a note on cholecystitis. What nutritional modifications are needed to control this condition?
5. Plan a day's diet for Anupma, a 32 years old working lady who has gall stones and is awaiting cholecystectomy.

12 Renal Disorders

The two kidneys lie to the sides of the upper abdomen, behind the intestines. In a normal human adult, each kidney is about 12 cm long, about 5 cm thick and weighs nearly 150 grams. Each kidney is about the size of a large orange, but bean-shaped. Kidneys are surrounded by two fat layers, which help to cushion it. The right kidney is slightly lower than the left kidney. In the outer part of the kidneys, tiny blood vessels cluster together to form structures called **glomeruli**. Each glomerulus acts as a filter. Filtration takes place through the semi permeable walls of the glomerular capillaries, which are almost impermeable to proteins and large molecules. The filtrate is thus virtually free of protein and has no cellular elements. About 20 percent of renal plasma flow is filtered each minute, which is known as **glomerular filtration rate** (GFR). The structure of the glomerulus allows waste products, some water and salt to pass into a tubule while keeping blood cells and protein in the bloodstream. Each glomerulus and tubule together is called '**nephron**' and the tubule comprises of proximal tubule, the loop of Henle, and the distal tubule, which finally empties into the collecting duct.

As the waste products and water passes along the tubule, some water and salts may be absorbed back into the bloodstream, depending on the current level of water and salt in the blood.

The liquid that remains at the end of each tubule is called **urine.** This drains into larger channels (ducts), which drain into the renal pelvis (the inner part of the kidney). From the renal pelvis, the urine passes down through ureter to the urinary bladder. Whereas, the filtered blood from each kidney collects into a large renal vein, which takes the blood back towards the heart.

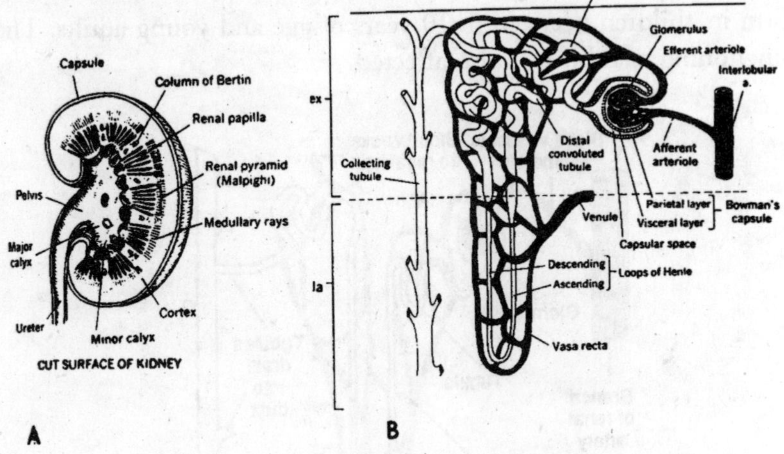

Source: Pansky B., Page-479

Normal composition of Urine	
Water	1.4 l/day
Urea	18.2 g/l
Uric acid	0.42 to 0.8 g/l
Creatinine	1 to 1.96 g/l
Ammonia	0.3 to 1 g/l
Minerals	0.32 eq/l
Calcium	10 to 300 mg
Na +	3 to 6 g/l
K+	2 to 4 g/l
Albumin	Nil
Bile	Nil
Sugar	Nil

Glomerulonephritis

Glomerulonephritis, also called nephritis, is a primary or secondary autoimmune renal disease characterized by inflammation of the glomeruli. In glomerulonephritis progressive loss of kidney function occurs over weeks to months. It is the most common in its acute form in children between 3–10 years of age and young adults. The functioning of tubules is also affected.

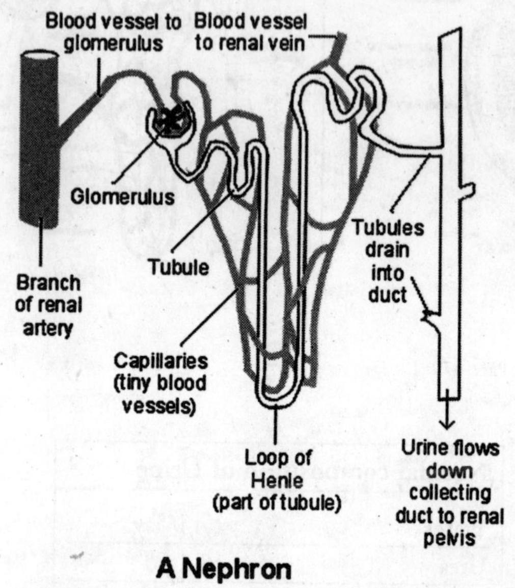

A Nephron

Causes

- The disease may be caused by specific problems with the body's immune system.
- Post-streptococcal glomerulonephritis: Glomerulonephritis may develop after a streptococcal infection in the throat or rarely in the skin.
- Viral infections: Among the virus that may trigger glomerulonephritis are the human immunodeficiency virus (HIV), which causes AIDS, and the hepatitis B and hepatitis C viruses, which affect the liver and can lead to chronic diseases.

Clinical Symptoms

The clinical symptoms of glomerulonephritis are given below:

- **Haematuria**—abnormal presence of blood in urine

- **Proteinuria**—an abnormal excess of serum proteins in the urine
- **Oedema**—excess accumulation of fluid in the body tissues
- **Hypertension**—high blood pressure
- Shortness of breath
- **Anorexia**—loss of appetite
- **Oliguria**—excretion of small amounts of urine in relation to fluid intake
- **Anuria**—an absence of urine production

Typical symptoms of glomerulonephritis are haematuria and proteinuria. Renal blood flow and glomerular filtration rate are reduced by as much as 50 percent or more and the damaged glomerular capillaries allow the plasma proteins and blood cells to pass through into the Bowman's capsule. The urine volume falls to between 500 to 1000 ml/day and sodium excretion is greatly reduced.

Urea and **creatinine** concentrations in plasma rise in proportion to the fall in glomerular filtration rate. The patient is generally anorexic. Vomiting may also occur, contributing to feeding problems. If the disease progresses to renal insufficiency, oliguria or anuria results, which is a signal for the development of acute renal failure.

Dietary Modifications

The main aim is to provide overall optimum nutrition. Adequate protein is given, unless oliguria or anuria develops. Salt is usually restricted as oedema and hypertension are common in this disease. Diet modifications are not strict or rigid. Bed rest and antibiotic therapy are mainly important. Fluid intake is adjusted according to the fluid output, which occurs through urine, vomiting or diarrhoea. As the disease progresses, the treatment becomes more defined.

Mostly the treatment involves bed rest, antibiotics to control infection, drugs to control hypertension and diuretics are often used to increase urine output. Dietary management plays an important role in the treatment.

The major objectives of dietary modification are:

- To maintain adequate and optimum nutrition.
- To give rest to the diseased kidney
- To prevent oedema and uraemia
- To achieve the above objectives, following dietary modifications are made:

Energy

Energy requirements are usually the same as in good health. For children 80 kcal/kg of body weight and 10 percent for infection is suggested. Sufficient calories are given. But if the patient is not suffering from any kind of malnutrition and is at bed rest since long time 10 to 20 percent calories can be reduced. Cereals in all forms are allowed.

Carbohydrates

Carbohydrate intake is liberal in order to provide sufficient kilocalories for energy needs. Carbohydrates help in protein sparing action, reduce catabolism of protein as well as prevent ketosis. Both simple carbohydrates such as sugars as well as complex form such as starches can be included in the diet.

Fats

Fat is not restricted. Emulsified and easily digestible fats are included. These give non-protein calories for energy needs, reduce the bulk of the diet and make the diet more palatable.

Proteins

If blood urea nitrogen is elevated and oliguria is present, dietary protein must be restricted. Usually the diet contains 0.5 to 0.6 g of protein/kg ideal body weight. If anuria develops, proteins should be stopped.

An intake of 20 to 40 g/day is considered sufficient. Pulses and groundnuts increase the urea levels in blood so these should be restricted. Rice is good as it has low amount of protein but of better quality than wheat. Sago can be included, as it does not contribute to protein. Fruits and vegetables, which are low in protein, sodium, and potassium can be given.

Sodium

The restriction of sodium varies with the degree of oliguria, oedema and hypertension. Usually the sodium is restricted to 500 to 1000 mg/day. With recovery, sodium intake can be increased.

Fluids

Fluid intake is adjusted according to the urine output. In the early stages of treatment, the fluid is usually decreased to allow the dispersal of fluid, which is accumulated in the body. Daily weighing is needed to monitor overall fluid balance. In later stages, the fluid intake is based on the volume of fluid excreted and an allowance of 500 ml/day is given for insensible water loss. Daily fluid replacement should be 500 ml plus daily amount excreted in the urine.

Nephrotic Syndrome

Nephrotic syndrome is a group of symptoms including protein in the urine (exceeding 3.5 grams per day), low blood protein levels, high cholesterol levels, and swelling due to water accumulation (oedema). In nephrotic syndrome, the urine contains large amounts of protein.

Causes of Nephrotic Syndrome

- Many times glomerulonephritis, progresses to nephrotic syndrome.
- Kidney disease caused by the diabetes can lead to nephrotic syndrome.
- Drugs such as gold or penicillamine can also cause it.
- Nephrotic syndrome can affect all age groups. In children, it is most common from age 2 to 6. This disorder occurs slightly more often in males than females.

Symptoms

- Proteinuria—an abnormal excess of serum proteins in the urine
- Swollen abdomen
- Swelling in the face
- Foamy appearance of the urine
- Weight gain because of fluid retention
- Loss of appetite
- High blood pressure
- Low level of albumin in the blood
- Tiredness and lethargy
- Oedema—excess accumulation of fluid in the body tissues

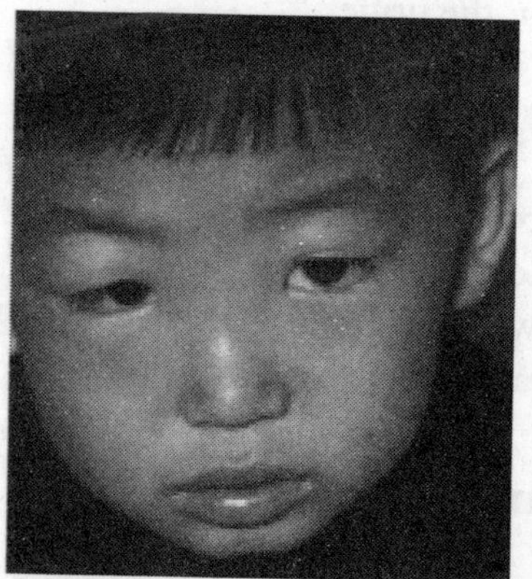
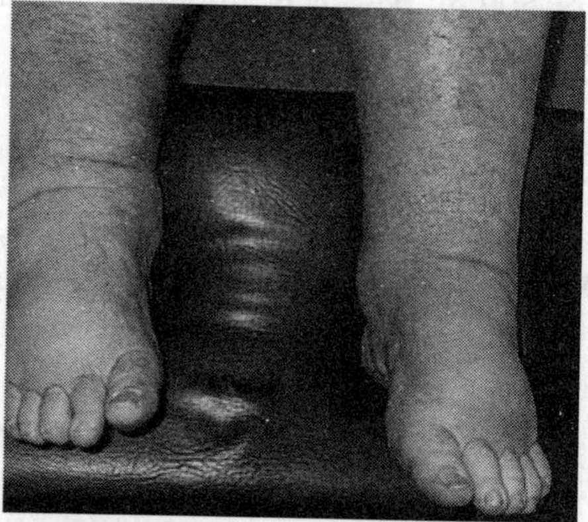

Pictures showing Oedema

In severe cases of nephrotic syndrome, the oedema can become extensive. Fluid may accumulate in the lower back, the arms, in the abdominal cavity (ascites) or in the chest between the lungs and the chest wall.

The main reason of fluid leak out from the blood vessels and into the body's tissues is low level of protein in the blood with nephrotic syndrome. As protein is lost from the body in the urine, the body makes more protein in the liver, which passes into the bloodstream. However, the amount made by the liver cannot keep up with the amount lost by the leaky kidneys, and so the blood level of protein goes down. When the blood level of protein is low then fluid tends to leak out of the blood vessels into the body tissues (*protein and other chemicals in the blood exert an 'osmotic pressure', which tends to pull fluid into the blood vessels. If the concentration of protein reduces, the osmotic pressure reduces, and fluid leaks out.*)

If the nephrotic syndrome persists for a long time then wasting of the muscles start. Depending on the cause of the nephrotic syndrome, one may also have other associated symptoms. For example, if someone has nephrotic syndrome due to diabetes, he/she may have a range of other symptoms caused by the diabetes.

Low albumin in the blood causes fluid to move from the blood into the tissue, causing swelling. The kidney perceives the decrease of fluid in the blood and aggressively retains as much fluid and salt as it can. This contributes to the body's fluid-overload state.

Complications

The main possible complications caused by nephrotic syndrome are due to the loss of normal proteins from the blood. These are as follows:

- An increased risk of developing infections. The first signs of infection (sore throat, fever, etc) should be taken seriously.
- An increased risk of developing blood clots in the blood vessels. In particular, a deep vein thrombosis in the legs. This can cause pain, swelling and other complications.
- A high cholesterol level. If this persists long-term it is a risk factor for developing heart disease.

Diagnosis of Disease

Urine Test—A simple 'dipstick' test of urine can confirm that it contains a lot of protein. The amount of protein lost can be measured by more detailed urine test.

Blood Test—Blood tests are done to identify the cause of the nephrotic syndrome.

Kidney Biopsy—When a small sample of tissue is removed from a kidney for clinical tests is known as kidney biopsy. The sample is looked at under a microscope, or tested in other ways. This is often the most important test to clarify the cause of a kidney problem, and its severity. Kidney biopsy is commonly done in many cases.

Treatment

Treatment of Oedema

Diuretics ('water tablets') help to rectify the problem of oedema. Diuretics work by acting on the cells in the kidney tubules to make them pass out more water rather than 'reabsorbing' water back into the bloodstream. Therefore, one passes out more urine. The excess fluid in the body's tissues then passes back into the bloodstream to keep the blood volume up to normal.

Dietary Modification

A high energy, low to moderate protein and fat and low sodium diet is prescribed.

Energy

A high energy diet must be provided for the efficient utilization of protein for tissue synthesis. High daily intakes of 50 to 60 kcal/kg of body weight are required.

Protein

Restriction of protein is usually done as increased protein intake may have an adverse effect on the functioning of the kidneys. The plasma albumin levels may have been reduced and it is the major cause of the development of oedema. Because of these reasons moderate to high protein intake is suggested according to the condition of the patient. A daily protein intake of 0.6 to 2 g per kg of body weight is recommended to replenish the depleted stores and to enhance the synthesis of albumin.

Sodium

Sodium levels in the diet must be sufficiently reduced to combat the massive oedema. Diuretics are also used to prevent further accumulation of fluid for some patients. For these patients, extreme degree of salt restriction is not required.

Acute Renal Failure (ARF)

Sudden and severe decrease in kidney function that is short term is known as acute renal failure. Renal function may stop suddenly because of some metabolic changes or injury, which causes life-threatening situation. Acute renal failure occurs when there is accumulation of high levels of waste products of the body's metabolism in the blood. ARF occurs when the kidneys are unable to excrete the daily load of toxins in the urine.

Patients with ARF are separated into two groups based on the amount of urine that is excreted out in a 24 hour period.

Oliguric—Patients who excrete less than 500 ml per day.

Nonoliguric—Patients who excrete more than 500 ml per day.

Causes

- Infectious diseases.
- Drug reactions in allergic or sensitive persons.
- Loss of blood during injury, accident, ulcers or at the time of delivery.
- Loss of fluid in diarrhoea, vomiting, diabetic coma (excessive urination and excessive sweating).
- Acute haemolytic disease when RBC's are destroyed due to some disease.
- Nephritis or Nephrosis can also result in acute renal failure.

Symptoms

- Anuria and oliguria are common in acute renal failure. The urinary output may be very low.
- Blood pressure may also rise.
- Serum urea nitrogen and creatinine levels are increased. Waste products of protein metabolism start accumulating in the blood.
- There is rise in serum potassium due to breakdown of tissue protein for providing energy.

Dietary Management

Energy

Non-protein sources of energy should be included. A minimum intake of 800 to1200 kcal of energy is required depending upon the condition of the patient.

Protein

In the initial stages, no protein is given to the patient. As the condition improves, only 15 to 25 g protein daily should be given to cover for endogenous losses. Complete proteins of high biological value should be included.

Fluid

According to the urine output and other additional losses from vomiting or diarrhoea, the fluid intake is adjusted. Fluid intake is usually restricted to 500 ml/day for an average adult with additions made for losses via other routes.

Chronic Renal Failure

Chronic renal failure represents a slow decline in kidney function over time. It may be caused by a number of disorders, which include long-standing hypertension, diabetes, congestive heart failure, sickle cell anaemia etc. If renal function declines to a very low level (end-stage renal disease) kidney dialysis may be necessary. A sudden decline in renal function may be triggered by a number of acute disease processes. Chronic renal failure also describes a progressive destruction of the basic units of the kidneys, the nephrons and may lead to total kidney failure. Chronic renal failure is also known as uraemia as the level of urea in blood is very high. Renal failure can result from a variety of systemic disorders.

When 90 percent of functioning renal tissue is destroyed uraemia occurs. It may be the end result of acute glomerulonephritis and nephrotic syndrome. Chronic renal failure is the final common pathway of many different diseases.

Causes

There are many causes of chronic renal failure which are as follows:

- Acute nephritis or nephrosis.
- Severe infections of the urinary tract.
- Kidney stones.
- High blood pressure.
- Polycystic diseases.
- Diabetes mellitus specially Type-1
- Gout
- Exposure to toxic substances

The urine volume depends upon GFR. Once chronic renal failure occurs, the normal functions of kidney like regulation of body fluids, electrolytes, pH and excretion of metabolites are disrupted and the disease occurs.

Clinical Symptoms

- Clinical symptoms include decreased renal blood flow and glomerular filtration rate.

- Sodium depletion, dehydration or water intoxication, increased susceptibility to infection etc.
- Oedema, high blood pressure, irregular heartbeats etc.
- Vomiting and hiccups.
- Neurological symptoms like peripheral neuropathy, twitching, convulsions and coma.
- Anaemia in many cases resulting in tiredness and breathlessness.
- Skin changes like pigmentation.

Dietary Management in Chronic Renal Failure

The objectives of dietary management in chronic renal failure are given below:

- To maintain electrolyte balance
- To prevent protein catabolism
- To control fluid and electrolyte losses from vomiting and diarrhoea
- To maintain optimal nutritional status
- To maintain appetite
- To control hypertension
- To retard progression of renal failure

Energy

Adequate kilocalories are mandatory. Carbohydrates and fats must supply sufficient non-protein kilocalories to spare protein for tissue protein synthesis and to supply energy. About 350 to 450 gm of carbohydrates should be provided to patient everyday. If the kilocalorie intake is inadequate, endogenous protein catabolism to supply energy will further increase or aggravate the problem of uraemia.

Protein

Protein intake can be reduced to 0.5 gm/kg of body weight per day. This helps to reduce azotemia and hyperkalemia. When blood urea nitrogen rises, the protein intake needs to be restricted to 15 to 20 gm/day. Protein restriction may not be necessary in the absence of symptoms in few cases. As renal failure progresses, the patient develop symptoms of uraemia and may be treated by regular haemodialysis or peritoneal dialysis or by renal transplantation.

Fluid

The fluid intake is monitored very carefully as there is a danger of both water intoxication from overloading as well as dehydration due to less water intake, as the capacity of failing kidneys, to handle water is limited. So depending upon the condition of the patient, the fluid intake is decided.

Sodium and Potassium

Sodium intake varies between 500 mg to 2 g per day. Whereas, the potassium intake is kept between 1500 to 2000 mg per day. Hypokalemia can occur at any time in chronic renal failure and in such cases small dose of potassium should be given with proper checking up of serum levels.

> Diuretics help the kidneys eliminate excess salt and water from the body's tissues and the blood. This helps reduce the swelling caused by fluid build-up in the tissues. The reduction of fluid dilates the walls of arteries and lowers blood pressure.

Dialysis

In the management of end stage of renal disease, dialysis is often used on temporary or permanent basis. The two major forms of dialysis are hemodialysis and peritoneal dialysis. In hemodialysis, the blood is sent through a filter that removes waste products. The clean blood is returned to the body. Hemodialysis is usually performed at a dialysis center three times per week for 3 to 4 hours.

In peritoneal dialysis, a fluid is put into the abdomen. This fluid captures the waste products from the blood. After few hours, the fluid

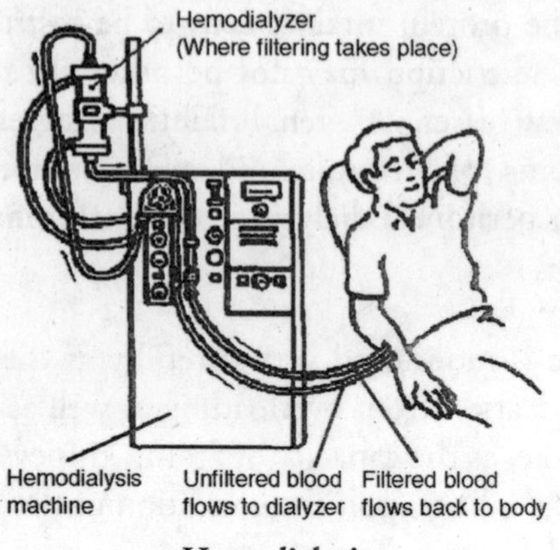

Hemodialysis

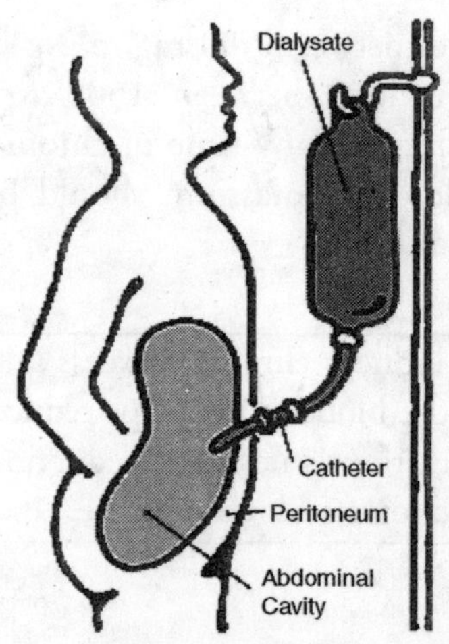

Peritoneal dialysis

containing the body's wastes is drained away. Then, a fresh bag of fluid is dripped into the abdomen. Patients can perform peritoneal dialysis themselves. Patients using continuous ambulatory peritoneal dialysis (CAPD) change fluid four times a day. Another form of peritoneal dialysis, called continuous cycling peritoneal dialysis (CCPD), can be performed at night with a machine that drains and refills the abdomen automatically.

Creatinine is produced from creatine, a molecule of major importance for energy production in muscles. Creatine is synthesized in the liver and utilized by the body to store energy. Creatine is sold as a dietary supplement and is used by athletes as a "legal steroid to increase muscle bulk. Creatinine, a waste product from protein in the diet and from the muscles of the body, is removed from the body by the kidneys, as kidney disease progresses, the level of creatinine in the blood increases. Approximately 2 percent of the body's creatine is converted to creatinine every day. Creatinine is transported through the bloodstream to the kidneys. The kidneys filter out most of the creatinine and dispose of it in the urine. The kidneys maintain the blood creatinine in a normal range. Creatinine has been found to be a fairly reliable indicator of renal functioning. Abnormally high levels of creatinine warn of possible malfunction or failure of the kidneys, sometimes even before a patient reports any symptoms. It is for this reason that standard blood and urine tests routinely check the amount of creatinine in the blood.

- Creatinine can also increase temporarily as a result of muscle injury.
- Creatinine levels are generally slightly lower during pregnancy.

Muscular young or middle-aged adults may have more creatinine in their blood than the general population. Infants have normal levels of about 0.2 or more, depending on their muscle development. A person with only one kidney may have a normal level of about 1.8 or 1.9. Creatinine levels that reach 2.0 or more in babies and 10.0 or more in adults may indicate the need for dialysis to remove wastes from the blood.

Review Questions

1. Discuss the role of kidneys in maintaining homeostasis in the body.
2. What is glomerulonephritis? Write down its dietary management.
3. Write down the difference between glomerulonephritis and nephritic syndrome.
4. Give the principal causes of acute renal failure.
5. When does a patient require kidney dialysis? Explain haemodialysis and peritoneal dialysis in brief.

Endocrine System Disorders

The endocrine system is a control system of ductless glands that secrete chemical "instant messengers" called hormones that circulate within the body via the bloodstream to affect distant cells within specific organs. Endocrine glands secrete their products immediately into the blood or interstitial fluid, without storage of the chemical. Hormones act as "messengers," and are carried by the bloodstream to different cells in the body, which interpret these messages and act on them. Endocrine glands include pituitary, thyroid, and adrenal glands, but not exocrine glands such as salivary glands, sweat glands and glands within the gastrointestinal tract.

Hypothalamus and Pituitary

The hypothalamus, a collection of specialized cells that is located in the lower central part of the brain, is the primary link between the endocrine and nervous systems. Nerve cells in the hypothalamus control the pituitary gland by producing chemicals that either stimulate or suppress hormone secretions from the pituitary.

Although it is no bigger than a pea, the pituitary gland, located at the base of the brain just beneath the hypothalamus, is considered the most important part of the endocrine system. It's often called the "master gland" because it makes hormones that control several other endocrine glands. The production and secretion of pituitary hormones can be influenced by factors such as emotions and seasonal changes. To accomplish this, the hypothalamus relays information sensed by the brain (such as environmental temperature, light exposure patterns, and feelings) to the pituitary.

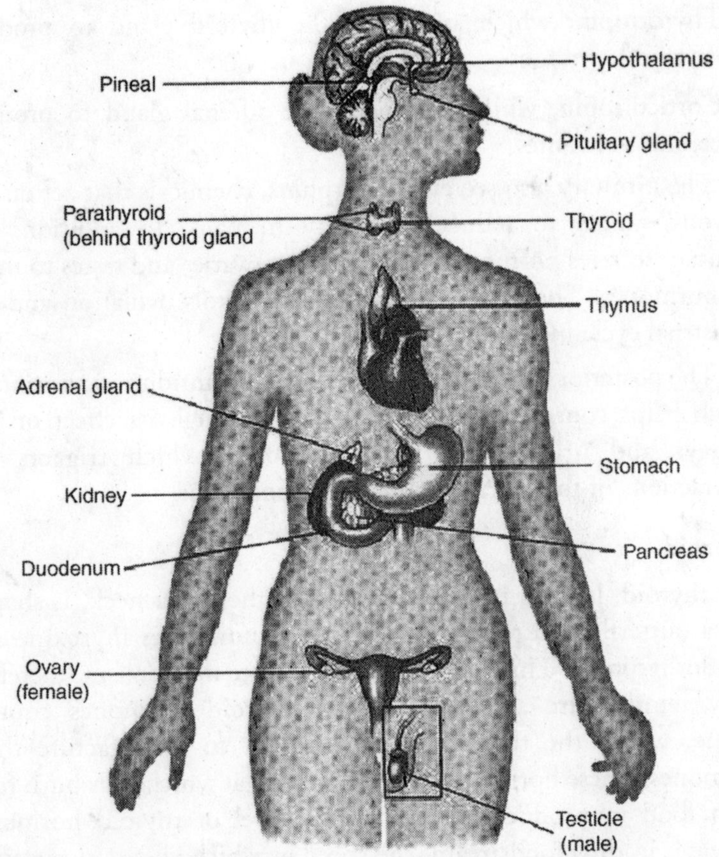

Hormones secreted by the endocrine glands

The tiny pituitary is divided into two parts: the anterior lobe and the posterior lobe. The anterior lobe regulates the activity of the thyroid, adrenals, and reproductive glands. Among the hormones it produces are:

- Growth hormone, which stimulates the growth of bone and other body tissues and plays a role in the body's handling of nutrients and minerals
- Prolactin, which activates milk production in women who are breastfeeding

- Thyrotropin, which stimulates the thyroid gland to produce thyroid hormones
- Corticotropin, which stimulates the adrenal gland to produce certain hormones

The pituitary also secretes endorphins, chemicals that act on the nervous system to reduce sensitivity to pain. In addition, the pituitary secretes hormones that signal the ovaries and testes to make sex hormones. The pituitary gland also controls ovulation and the menstrual cycle in women.

The posterior lobe of the pituitary releases antidiuretic hormone, which helps control body water balance through its effect on the kidneys and urine output, and oxytocin, which triggers the contractions of the uterus that occur during labor.

Thyroid

The thyroid, located in the front part of the lower neck, is shaped like a butterfly and produces the thyroid hormones thyroxine and triiodothyronine. Thyroid hormones regulate metabolism, therefore body temperature and weight. The thyroid hormones contain iodine, which the thyroid needs in order to manufacture these hormones. These hormones control the rate at which cells burn fuels from food to produce energy. As the level of thyroid hormones increases in the bloodstream, the speed at which chemical reactions occur in the body also increases. Thyroid hormones also play a key role in bone growth and the development of the brain and nervous system in children. The production and release of thyroid hormones is controlled by thyrotropin, which is secreted by the pituitary gland.

Parathyroid

Attached to the thyroid are four tiny glands that function together called the parathyroids. They release parathyroid hormone (PTH), which regulates the level of calcium in the blood with the help of calcitonin, which is produced in the thyroid. Both calcitonin and PTH control calcium metabolism, but their action is antagonist.

- When the Ca^{2+} in the blood rises, less PTH and more calcitonin is secreted.
- When the Ca^{2+} in the blood falls, more PTH and less calcitonin is secreted.

Adrenal

The body has two triangular adrenal glands, one on top of each kidney. The adrenal glands have two parts, each of which produces a set of hormones and has a different function. The outer part, the adrenal cortex, produces hormones called corticosteroids that influence or regulate salt and water balance in the body, the body's response to stress, metabolism, the immune system, and sexual development and function. The inner part, the adrenal medulla, produces catecholamines, such as epinephrine. Also called adrenaline, epinephrine increases blood pressure and heart rate when the body experiences stress.

Pineal

The pineal body, also called the pineal gland, is located in the middle of the brain. It secretes melatonin, a hormone that may help regulate the wake-sleep cycle.

Pancreas

The pancreas produces mainly two important hormones, insulin and glucagon. These are secreted by Islets of Langerhans. They work together to maintain a steady level of glucose, or sugar, in the blood and to keep the body supplied with fuel to produce and maintain stores of energy.

Glucagon—Increases the blood sugar level by speeding up the breakdown of glycogen into glucose in the liver and releasing it into the blood.

Insulin—Lowers the blood sugar level by accelerating transport of glucose to cells and converting glucose to glycogen.

Gonads

The gonads are the main source of sex hormones. In males, they are located in the scrotum. Male gonads, or testes, secrete hormones called androgens, the most important of which is testosterone. These hormones regulate body changes associated with sexual development, including enlargement of the penis, the growth spurt that occurs during puberty, and the appearance of other male secondary sex characteristics such as deepening of the voice, growth of facial and pubic hair, and the increase in muscle growth and strength. Working with hormones from the pituitary gland, testosterone also supports the production of sperm by the testes.

The female gonads, the ovaries, are located in the pelvis. They produce eggs and secrete the female hormones estrogen and progesterone. Estrogen is involved in the development of female sexual features such as breast growth, the accumulation of body fat around the hips and thighs, and the growth spurt that occurs during puberty. Both estrogen and progesterone are also involved in pregnancy and the regulation of the menstrual cycle.

Diabetes

Diabetes (medically known as diabetes mellitus) is the name given to a disorder in which the body has problems in the regulation of blood glucose, or blood sugar, levels. The full name 'diabetes mellitus' is derived from the Greek word 'diabetes' meaning siphon—to pass through, and 'mellitus,' the Latin word for sweet. It is a group of metabolic diseases characterized by hyperglycemia (excess blood glucose) resulting from defects in insulin secretion, insulin action or both. The disease is chronic and affects the metabolism of carbohydrate, protein, fat, water and electrolytes.

Sources of Blood Glucose

- Diet
- Glycogen

Normal blood sugar control

In the body, glucose is converted into energy. Blood contains some glucose (sugar). The liver is also able to manufacture glucose. Too much sugar in the blood is not good for the health. The body changes most of the food into sugar. Under normal circumstances the hormone insulin, which is made by the beta cells of the islets of Langerhans of the pancreas, carefully regulates glucose present in the blood. Insulin stimulates cells to absorb enough glucose from the blood for the energy, or fuel, that they need. Insulin also stimulates the liver to absorb and store any glucose that's left over. After a meal the amount of glucose in the blood rises, and this triggers the release of insulin. When blood glucose levels fall, for example during exercise, insulin levels fall too. A second hormone manufactured by the pancreas is called glucagon. It stimulates the liver to release glucose when it's needed, and this raises the level of glucose in the blood.

Insulin cannot be taken as a pill because the digestive juices in the stomach destroy insulin before it starts working.

If the body does not make enough insulin or the insulin does not work properly, blood glucose level increases leading to diabetes. Diabetes can lead to blindness, heart disease, stroke, kidney failure, amputations (having a toe or foot removed), and nerve damage. In women, diabetes can cause problems during pregnancy and make it more likely that the baby will be born with birth defects.

Pre-diabetes means that the blood sugar is higher than normal but lower than the diabetes range. It also means that the person is at risk of getting type 2 diabetes and heart diseases.

Symptoms

The symptoms of diabetes can develop gradually and may be hard to identify at first.

The classic symptoms of diabetes are:

- Hyperglycemia
- Frequent urination, with large volumes of urine (polyuria)
- Excessive thirst (polydipsia)
- Hunger (polyphagia)

- Dehydration
- Fatigue
- Weight loss

Symptoms of Type 1 Diabetes	Symptoms of Type 2 Diabetes
Increased thirst	Increased thirst
Increased urination	Increased urination
Weight loss in spite of increased appetite	Increased appetite
Fatigue	Fatigue
Nausea	Blurred vision
Vomiting	Slow-healing infections and impotence in men in some cases

Other symptoms might include:

- Dry or itchy skin
- Impotence (in a male)
- Vaginal yeast infections (in a female)
- Poor healing of cuts and scrapes
- Excessive or unusual infections
- Fatigue
- Blurry vision
- Odd aches and pains
- Dry mouth

Diabetes affects the way body uses blood sugar. Even when someone eats as much as usual, he/she may loose weight if muscle tissues don't get enough glucose to generate growth and energy. This is the reason why type I diabetics usually loose weight.

There are many risk factors for diabetes, which include:

- A parent, brother, or sister with diabetes
- Obesity
- Age greater than 45 years
- Gestational diabetes or delivering a baby weighing more than 9 pounds
- High blood pressure
- High blood levels of triglycerides
- High blood cholesterol level

Types of Diabetes

- Type 1 (insulin dependent results from β cells destruction)
- Type 2 (non-insulin dependent).
- Gestational diabetes (during pregnancy).

Type 1 Diabetes

Type 1 diabetes, or insulin-dependent diabetes, has traditionally been termed "juvenile diabetes" because it represents a majority of cases of diabetes affecting children. Type 1 diabetes is caused by an autoimmune disorder—a problem with the body's immune system. In a healthy body, beta cells of the islets of Langerhans in the pancreas make insulin. Insulin is a hormone that allows the body to use energy from food. With this form of diabetes, the beta cells of the pancreas no longer make insulin because the body's immune system has attacked and destroyed them. When enough beta cells are destroyed, symptoms of diabetes appear. The principal treatment of type 1 diabetes, even for the earliest stages, is replacement of insulin. Without insulin, ketosis and diabetic ketoacidosis can develop which further lead to coma or death.

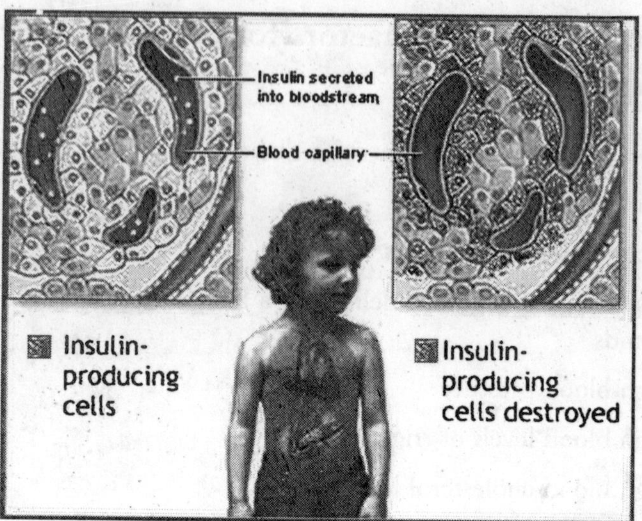

Diagram showing Type I diabetes

Type 2 Diabetes is also known as "non insulin-dependent diabetes mellitus" (NIDDM) or "adult-onset diabetes." Type 2 diabetes is the most common form of diabetes mellitus. About 90 to 95 percent of people have this type of diabetes. People with type 2 diabetes produce insulin, but either does not make enough insulin or their bodies do not use the insulin they make. Most of the people who have this type of diabetes are overweight. People can develop type 2 diabetes at any age, even during childhood. This form of diabetes usually begins with insulin resistance, a condition in which fat, muscle, and liver cells do not use insulin properly. At first, the pancreas keeps up with the added demand by producing more insulin in time. However, further it loses the ability to secrete enough insulin in response to meals. Being overweight and inactive increases the chances of developing type 2 diabetes.

In type 1 diabetes, the immune system mistakes beta cells for invaders and attacks them. Treatment for type 1 diabetes includes taking insulin, making wise food choices, being physically active, and controlling blood pressure and cholesterol.

Gestational Diabetes

Gestational diabetes (also called glucose intolerance of pregnancy) is a temporary condition that occurs during pregnancy. It affects two to four per cent of all pregnancies and involves an increased risk of developing diabetes for both mother and child. Some women develop gestational diabetes during the late stages of pregnancy. Although this form of diabetes usually goes away after the baby is born, a woman who has had it is more likely to develop type 2 diabetes later in life. The hormones of pregnancy or a shortage of insulin causes gestational diabetes.

Causes of Gestational Diabetes

- A family history of diabetes in parents or siblings
- Gestational diabetes in a previous pregnancy
- The presence of a birth defect in a previous pregnancy
- Obesity in the woman, BMI greater than 29
- Older maternal age (over the age of 30)
- Previous stillbirth or spontaneous miscarriage
- A previous delivery of a large baby (greater than 9 pounds)
- A history of pregnancy induced high blood pressure, urinary tract infections, hydramnios (extra amniotic fluid), etc.
- A history of polycystic ovary syndrome
- Hirsutism (excessive body and facial hair)

Risk for babies born to mothers with Gestational Diabetes

- Large, fat baby
- Birth trauma
- Neonatal hypoglycemia (low blood sugar in the newborn)
- Prolonged newborn jaundice
- Low blood calcium
- Respiratory distress syndrome

Diabetes is derived from the Greek verb diabainein, which means to stand with legs apart, as in urination. Diabetes mellitus means, honey-sweet urine. Whereas, diabetes insipidus means bland or insipid urine which is caused by the undersecretion of vasopressin also known as antidiuretic hormone (ADH) that controls water metabolism. ADH is made in the hypothalamus and is stored and secreted by the posterior pituitary gland.

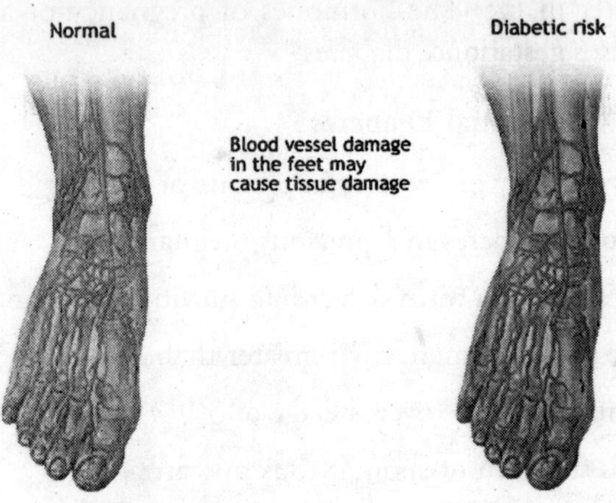

Diabetic blood circulation in foot

Diagnosis of Diabetes

- Fasting blood glucose level
- Non fasting blood glucose level
- Oral glucose tolerance test
- Urine analysis (glycosuria and Ketonuria)

Blood Glucose (g /dl)	
	Fasting
Normal	<100
Diabetic	>140
Impaired glucose tolerance	100-140

Ketones are produced by the breakdown of fat and muscle, they are toxic at high levels. Ketones in the blood cause a condition called "acidosis" (low blood pH). Urine test, detects both glucose and ketones in the urine.

Patients with type 1 diabetes usually develop symptoms over a short period of time, and the condition is often diagnosed in an emergency setting. In addition to having high glucose levels, acutely ill type 1 diabetics have high levels of ketones.

Complications

The complications are far less common and less severe in people who have well-controlled blood sugar levels. In fact, the better the control, the lower the risk of complications. Hence patient education, understanding and participation is vital. Acute and chronic complications of diabetes are as follows.

Acute

- Diabetic ketoacidosis
- Hypoglycemia
- Diabetic coma

Chronic

Microvascular disease (due to damage to small blood vessels)

Dietary management—Dietary control is an integral part of management for the diabetic. The diet should always provide the essentials of good nutrition and adjustments must be made from time to time for changing metabolic needs.

The mainstays of treatment are:

1. Working towards obtaining ideal body weight
2. Following a diabetic diet

3. Regular exercise
4. Diabetic medication if needed

Calories—Patients with Type 1 diabetes should have a diet that has approximately 35 calories per kg of body weight per day. Patients with Type 2 diabetes generally are put on a 1500–1800 kcal per day to promote weight loss and maintenance of ideal body weight. However, this may vary depending on the person's age, sex, activity level, current weight and body style. Men have more muscle mass in general and therefore may require more calories. Muscle burns more calories per hour than fat. Also, people whose activity level is low will have less daily caloric needs.

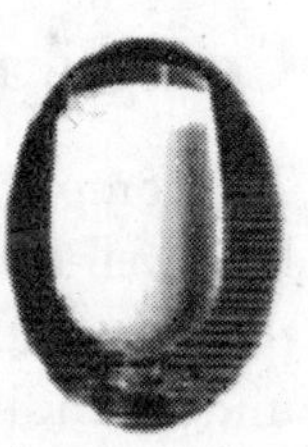

Proteins—Since diabetics in general are in negative nitrogen balance as large quantities of nitrogen are excreted in the urine, they should receive about twice as much protein as normal subjects. The proteins should be of high biological value and provide about 20–25 percent of the calories in the diet. A diet high in protein is good for diabetics because

1. It supplies the essential amino acids needed for tissue repair.
2. Protein does not raise the blood sugar during absorption, as do carbohydrates.

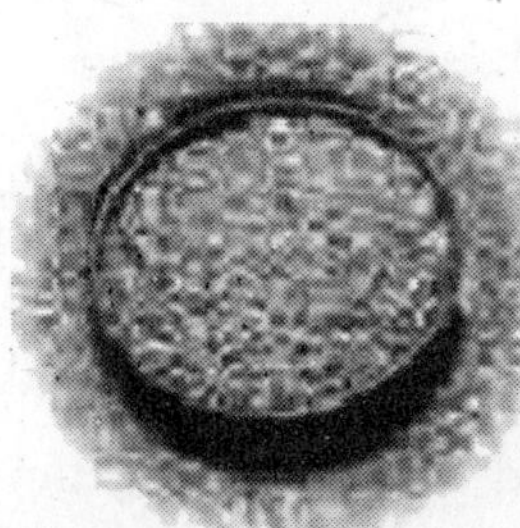

3. It does not supply more of calories.

Carbohydrates—Generally, carbohydrates should make up about 40 to 50 percent of the daily calories. In general, lower carbohydrate intake is associated with lower sugar levels in the blood but many studies have shown that raising the carbohydrate intake does not adversely affect blood glucose levels, glucose tolerance, or insulin requirements provided that total calories are not increased. Inspite of high carbohydrate along with high fibre improves insulin functioning. Simple carbohydrates (mono and disaccharides) like sweets, chocolates should be avoided. The daily intake of carbohydrate should provide about 40 percent of the calories to prevent ketosis.

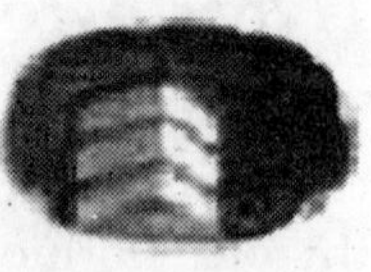

Fats—The fat allowance makes up the remaining calories for most diets after protein and carbohydrate intakes have been established. Fat intake is lowered to 20 percent or less of the days energy intake in case of adult diabetics, who are also obese. Foods high in saturated fat and cholesterol are limited.

Fibre—Soluble fibre in oat bran, legumes (dried beans of all kinds, peas and lentils), and pectin (from fruit, such as apples) and forms in root vegetables (such as carrots) is considered especially helpful for people with either form of diabetes. Soluble fibre helps control blood sugar by delaying gastric (stomach) emptying, retarding the entry of glucose into the bloodstream and lessening the postprandial (post-meal) rise in blood sugar. It may lessen insulin requirements in those with type 1 diabetes. Because fibre slows the digestion of foods, it can help stop the sudden rise in blood glucose that may occur after a low-fibre meal. Such blood sugar peaks stimulate the pancreas to pump out more insulin.

One can reduce the risk of getting diabetes and even return to normal blood sugar levels with modest weight loss and moderate physical activity.

Planning the Diet

1. Avoid roots and tubers e.g. potato, sweet potato, colocasia, yam, tapioca except carrot and radish.
2. Avoid sugar, glucose, jams, jaggery, honey, sweets, nuts, horlicks, bournvita, etc.
3. Avoid fried foods.
4. Include salads but no salad dressing like mayonnaise.
5. Include plenty of green leafy vegetables.
6. Excess of fats and oils should be restricted.
7. Food exchanges should be used.
8. Avoid alcohol.
9. Include high fibre foods.
10. Avoid fruits such as mango, banana, chickoo, custard apple etc.

Hyperthyroidism and Hypothyroidism

The thyroid gland is one of the seven major glands that make up the endocrine system. The thyroid gland manufactures and secretes thyroid hormone that greatly influences many body activities. Thyroid hormone controls basal metabolic rate by catalyzing the oxidative processes in cells. Diseases of the thyroid gland produce too much or too little thyroid hormone; consequently, the effects of thyroid diseases fall into two general categories: hyperthyroidism or **hypothyroidism.**

Supplementation of the diet with zinc improves the thyroid function

Causes of Thyroid Diseases

There are a variety of factors, which can contribute to the development of thyroid problems:

- Too much or shortage of iodine in the diet.
- Excessive consumption of some soy products such as soy protein capsules and powders.
- Radiation treatment to the head, neck or chest. Radiation treatment for tonsils, lymph nodes, thymus gland problems or acne.
- Over-consumption of uncooked 'goitrogenic' foods such as brussel sprouts, broccoli, turnip, radish, cauliflower, cabbage and kale.

Iodine is necessary for the synthesis of the thyroid hormones triiodothyronine and thyroxine (T3 and T4). In conditions producing endemic goitre, when iodine is not available, these hormones cannot be made. In response to low thyroid hormones, the pituitary gland releases thyroid stimulating hormone (TSH). Thyroid stimulating hormone acts to increase synthesis of T3 and T4, but in excess it also causes the thyroid gland to grow as it attempts to comply with the pituitary's demands. Apart from iodine deficiency, other causes of goiter involve conditions of the thyroid—such as nodules, cancer, hyperthyroidism and hypothyroidism.

Contd..

A generally accepted desirable dietary iodine intake by an adult is 100-300 mcg/day. The average daily salt intake in India is 10 g. From the average daily intake of 10 g iodine fortified salt, the estimated availability of iodine would be 150 mcg, of which about 30 percent is lost during cooking. The remaining 105 mcg is ingested and from this about 70 percent is absorbed by the body. This means approximately only 73.5 mcg is absorbed per day from iodine fortified salt.

Thyroid Diseases

Hyperthyroidism–Grave's disease

Hypothyroidism–Myxoedema, creatinism

Hyperthyroidism

Hyperthyroidism is characterized by an overactive thyroid gland and increased circulating levels of thyroid hormone. In general, hyperthyroidism is more common in young adults between the age of 20 and 40, and is found more often in women than in men.

Clinically, the patient exhibits signs and symptoms such as

- Increased heart rate, commonly more than 100 beats a minute
- Increased blood pressure
- Moist skin
- Perspiration
- Nervousness
- Increased appetite
- Weight loss
- Insomnia
- Diarrhea
- Weakness

- Thickened skin
- Bulging eyes
- Confusion
- Tremor—usually a fine trembling in the hands and fingers
- An enlarged thyroid gland (goitre), which may appear as a swelling at the base of the neck

Enlargement of the thyroid gland and protrusion of the eyes are the two typical symptoms of hyperthyroidism. Hyperthyroidism should be treated as quickly as possible to avoid unnecessary stimulation to various system of the body. Hyperthyroidism is a fairly common condition. It is more common in women because a common form of hyperthyroidism is of autoimmune origin, and women are more commonly afflicted with autoimmune diseases than men. Graves' disease is caused by autoimmunity. The manifestations of Grave disease include:

1) Hyperthyroidism
2) Enlarged thyroid gland (goitre)
3) Protruding eyes.

Iodine deficiency and use of thyroid-stimulating foods or drugs are common causes of hyperthyroidism.

Hypothyroidism

Hypothyroidism arises when too little thyroid hormone is produced and circulated in the blood stream. This is caused by inflammation of the gland, autoimmune thyroiditis, or the wasting away of the gland itself. Thyroid problems could be due to an iodine deficient diet (iodine is an essential component of the thyroid hormones).

Regardless of the cause, patients with hypothyroidism share common signs and symptoms associated with the lack of thyroid hormone. These include

- Fatigue
- Lack of energy

- A dull facial expression
- Hoarse voice
- Droopy eyelids
- Puffy and swollen eyes and face
- Weight gain
- Constipation
- Aversion to cold
- Dry hair and skin
- Low body temperature
- Decreased heart rate and blood pressure.

Under secretion of thyroid causes myxoedema, creatinism and enlarged thyroid gland (goitre). Hypothyroidism is considerably less common than hyperthyroidism. It, like hyperthyroidism, is more common in women than in men. If it occurs in childhood, there can be severe developmental defects.

Hypothyroidism is usually caused because of the following reasons

- Destruction of the thyroid gland by surgery
- Non-development of the gland
- Radiation
- Drug therapy
- Iodine deficiencies in which thyroid hormone is not manufactured correctly
- Destruction of the functioning portion of the gland by goiter, inflammation, etc.

Myxoedema

Advanced hypothyroidism, known as myxoedema, is very rare. When it occurs, though, the condition can be life threatening. Its symptoms include:

- Drowsiness
- Intense intolerance to cold followed by profound lethargy and unconsciousness.

Thyroid under-secretion in adults causes facial oedema, coarse skin, decreased mental acuity and decreased metabolism. Myxoedema is defined as hypothyroidism acquired, not inherited in the adults.

Creatinism

Thyroid under-secretion in children may cause stunted growth, retarded mental development, and delayed bone and tooth deve-lopment. Early identification and replacement therapy may stop this condition.

Dietary Management of Hypothyroidism

Some foods, such as rapeseed (used to make canola oil) and brassica vegetables (cabbage, Brussel sprouts, broccoli, cauliflower, turnip) contain natural goitrogens which cause the thyroid gland to enlarge by interfering with the thyroid hormone synthesis. So these vegetables should be avoided. Other foods that have goitrogens include maize, millets, sorghum, sweet potatoes, soy and its products.

One should not have more than 25 to 30 gm of fat per day. Fat intake should come mainly from vegetable oils, which are rich in essential fatty acids.

Vitamin and mineral intake should meet the daily requirements.

Use very little sodium chloride (common salt). Avoid salted confectioneries, chips and pickles.

One should limit smoking, alcohol and caffeine (found in tea, coffee, cola and chocolate) as these can raise the metabolic rate.

Increase iodine consumption by eating the following:

- Seafood—fish, fresh and canned oysters, prawns, shrimps, mussels and seaweed. Try to eat fish three times a week.
- The iodine content of other foods such as cereals, fruits, vegetables, meat, milk and eggs depends on the iodine of the soil and water in the area where they have been cultivated. Food products cultivated along the coastline will contain more iodine than food grown at inland farms.

- Consume only iodized table salt.

The diet should be low in calorie, adequate protein, fat, minerals, and vitamins.

Dietary Management of Hyperthyroidism

Intake of Vitamin A, B complex and C should be increased to twice the daily requirement. The diet should include:

- A combination of pulses and wheat sprouts.
- Carotene rich foods like papaya, mango, fenugreek leaves and spinach.

During hyperthyroidism, calcium and phosphorous excretion is greatly increased. Hence, calcium and phosphorus rich food like milk, milk products (yoghurt and cottage cheese) and dark green leafy vegetables (spinach) must be consumed. Ragi prepared with milk is an excellent source of calcium and phosphorus.

The diet for hyperthyroidism consists of high calories, proteins, vitamins and minerals. The diet should consist of egg, meat, poultry and cereal and pulse combination.

A person suffering from hyperthyroidism should also limit smoking, alcohol, and caffeine containing beverages like tea, coffee, and chocolate etc.

Facts about Hyperthyroidism

- Hyperthyroidism is a medical condition characterized by an abnormally high level of thyroid hormone in the bloodstream.
- Hyperthyroidism is commonly referred to as "overactive thyroid."
- Hyperthyroidism is also known as thyrotoxicosis from the prefix "thyro-" meaning thyroid, the term "toxic" meaning poisonous, and the suffix "-osis" meaning condition.
- Symptoms of hyperthyroidism may include a rapid heartbeat, muscle weakness, tremor, weight loss, and the inability to tolerate heat.

- The most common form of hyperthyroidism is Graves disease. About 95 percent of affected individuals have this form of the disease.
- The three major treatment options-medication, radioactive iodine, and surgery-work by decreasing the amount of thyroid hormone produced. The goal of treatment is to bring the body into homeostasis or a healthy, balanced condition.
- About 30 percent of people with Graves' disease have associated eye disease. Hyperthyroid eye disease may cause significant changes in vision along with eyes that bulge or protrude from the face. Other problems with the eyes vary greatly and may include discomfort, pain, or excessive tearing to blurry vision or even double vision.

Polycystic Ovary Syndrome (PCOS)

PCOS is also known clinically as Stein-Leventhal syndrome.The ovaries are the main reproductive organs in women that produce the eggs or ova. Eggs grow, develop, and mature in the ovaries and then are released during ovulation. Polycystic ovary syndrome (PCOS) is a syndrome in which the ovaries are enlarged and have several fluid-filled sacs known as cysts. Ovarian cysts form on the ovaries when the follicles (sacs) on the ovary that contain the egg mature, but do not release the egg into the fallopian tube, where these are fertilized.

Polycystic ovaries are usually 1.5 to 3 times larger than normal ovaries. A woman can have one to many cysts, which look like a string of pearls. Women with PCOS may experience a number of other symptoms as well. PCOS is a leading cause of infertility and is

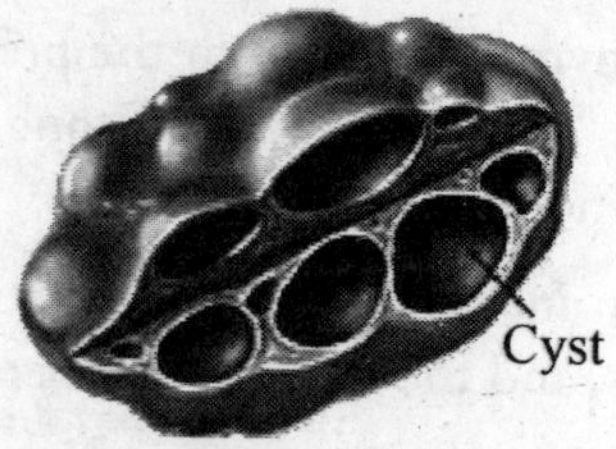

Polycystic Ovary

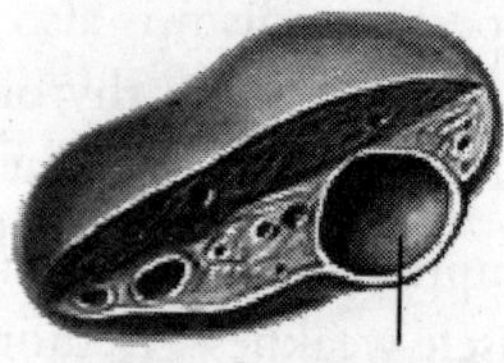

Normal Ovary

the most common reproductive syndrome in women of childbearing age (An estimated five to ten percent of women of childbearing age have PCOS (ages 20 to 40) and at least 30 percent of women have some symptoms of PCOS).

Causes of PCOS

The abnormal high levels of androgens (e.g., testosterone), the male hormones that are actually secreted in both men and women, trigger the problem. More production of androgen often results from overproduction of LH (luteinizing hormone), which is produced by the pituitary gland. When insulin levels in the blood are high enough, the ovary can be stimulated to produce more testosterone which prevents the ovaries from releasing an egg each month, causing infertility and menstrual irregularities. Obesity also causes insulin levels to rise and may thus intensify PCOS. Yet, not all women who are overweight develop PCOS. It appears to be an inherited condition.

- Genetic predisposition.
- Insulin resistance or hyperinsulinism (high blood levels of insulin).
- Obesity.
- Hyperandrogenism (excessive production of male hormones).
- Environmental chemical pollution (hormonal disruptors).

Symptoms of PCOS

Polycystic ovary syndrome is an endocrine (hormonal) disorder in which symptoms first appear in adolescence, around the start of menstruation. However, some women do not develop symptoms until their early to mid-20's. Although PCOS presents early in life, it persists through and beyond the reproductive years.

No two women experiencing PCOS have exactly the same symptoms. The following symptoms are very often associated with PCOS, but not all are seen in every woman:

1. Oligomenorrhoea—Infrequent menstrual periods, no menstrual periods, and/or irregular bleeding.
2. Amenorrhoea—Absence of menstruation.
3. Infrequent or no ovulation.
4. Increased serum levels of male hormones, such as testosterone.
5. Inability to get pregnant within six to 12 months of unprotected sexual intercourse (infertility).
6. Pelvic pain that lasts longer than six months.
7. Weight gain or obesity.
8. Diabetes, over-production of insulin, and inefficient use of insulin in the body.
9. Abnormal lipid levels (such as high or low cholesterol levels, and high triglycerides).
10. High blood pressure (over 140/90).
11. Hirsutism—Excess growth of hair on the face, chest, stomach, thumbs, or toes.
12. Male-pattern baldness or thinning hair.
13. Acne, oily skin, or dandruff.
14. Patches of thickened and dark brown or black skin on the neck, groin, underarms, or skin folds.
15. Skin tags, or tiny excess flaps of skin in the armpits or neck area.

PCOS is a health problem that can affect a woman's menstrual cycle, fertility, hormones, insulin production, heart, blood vessels, and appearance.

Women with PCOS have these characteristics

- High levels of male hormones, also called androgens
- An irregular or no menstrual cycle
- May or may not have many small cysts in their ovaries.

Recommended Nutrition Balance of Carbohydrates, Fats and Proteins

As a rough guide to overall nutritional intake, PCOS patients who are not obese are advised to eat about 50 percent of their calories in the form of healthy carbohydrates, 30 percent in the form of healthy fats and the balance in healthy protein. PCOS patients suffering from obesity should aim for about 50 percent of calories from carbohydrates, 30 percent protein and 20 percent fat.

Importance of Exercise

- Weight or strength training improves insulin resistance and metabolic rate.
- Regular aerobic exercise workouts benefit insulin resistance as well as a range of health indicators like serum cholesterol, blood pressure and cardiovascular function.
- All these benefits impact on polycystic ovary syndrome.
- Exercise on a regular basis.

The recommendations for the PCOS patient

- Try to select lower glycemic index foods as they will cause a slower rise in blood sugar. (Glycemic index is an indicator of how rapidly the food turns to sugar in the blood). The lower glycemic carbohydrates tend to have more fiber than the higher glycemic foods. For example, bran cereal (10 gm fibre/1/2 cup) has a lower glycemic index than cornflakes (1 gm fibre/1/2 cup). In other words, select breads, grains and cereals that are unprocessed.

- Adequate carbohydrate intake is must. Eating less than 40 grams of carbohydrate a day may induce ketosis.
- Avoid those carbohydrates that trigger more hunger or cravings (e.g. pasta triggers craving for some people).
- Vitamin and mineral supplements:
- Calcium 1000 mg–1500 mg
- Multivitamin with minerals
- Drink at least 8 cups of water as a low carbohydrate intake can cause dehydration.
- For heart health, limit foods high in saturated and trans fats (i.e. fatty red meat, whole milk dairy, butter and stick margarine, chicken skin, fried foods, rich desserts, etc.). Select mainly monounsaturated fats (i.e. olive oil, canola oil, nuts) and omega 3 fats (fatty fish such as salmon and bluefish, flaxseed, nuts) as these fats are heart healthy.

Menopause

Menopause is the end of menstruation. The time in a woman's life when monthly cycles of menstruation cease forever and the level of hormones produced by the ovaries decreases. The word comes from the Greek mens, meaning monthly, and pausis, meaning cessation. Menopause is part of a woman's natural aging process when her ovaries produce lower levels of the hormones estrogen and progesterone and when she is no longer able to become pregnant. Menopause usually occurs in the late 40s or early 50s, but it can also be brought about by surgical removal of both ovaries (oophorectomy), or by some chemotherapies that destroy ovarian function or when her ovaries stop functioning for any other reason. Perimenopause refers to the several years before menopause when a woman may begin experiencing the first signs of her menopausal transition. But many people use the term 'menopause' for both the perimenopausal years as well as the few years following menopause.

The most common signs of Menopause

Changing levels of estrogen and progesterone can cause a variety of symptoms. One may have little or no trouble with hot flashes or other signs of menopause. Some women, however, have slight discomfort or worse. Common changes someone might have are:

- Periods become irregular. Some women have short times of heavy bleeding. These are all fairly common. Very heavy bleeding for many days may occur.
- The hot flash is the best-known sign of menopause. Some women start getting hot flashes several years before their periods stop. During a hot flash one suddenly feels hot. It may begin with a sudden tingling in the fingers, toes, cheeks, or ears. Sometimes only certain parts of the body become red or flushed. The most common parts of the body to get fully flushed are the face and the neck. Each hot flash can last from 30 seconds to five minutes. Hot flashes happen because the body is making less estrogen, a female hormone.
- Tissues in the genital area become drier and thinner as estrogen levels change.
- Feeling tired is another common symptom. One might have trouble getting to sleep, waking early, or getting back to sleep after waking up in the middle of the night. Women may be awakened by night sweats and feel the need to go to the bathroom.
- Women usually become more moody, irritable, or depressed during the time of menopause. There is a connection between changes in the estrogen level and emotions. Other causes for these mood shifts might be stress, family changes such as children leaving home, and feeling tired.
- Visible changes during menopause include a thickening at the waist, loss of muscle mass and increase in fat tissue, or thinning and loss of stretchiness in the skin.

- The bones get weak and can break more easily.
- Many women also experience headaches, memory problems, joint and muscle stiffness or pain, sudden depression, forgetfulness, dizziness, thinning scalp hair and growth of facial hair.

As estrogen levels begin to decline, the levels of the harmful low-density lipoprotein (LDL) cholesterol begin to rise and the advantageous high-density lipoprotein (HDL) levels decrease. Risk of heart diseases increase.

Dietary Management of Menopause

- Increase daily intake of fruits and vegetables. Choose melons, bananas and citrus fruits like oranges and lemons, which are high in potassium. Potassium rich foods help balance sodium and water retention. In vegetables eat more of yam, dark leafy vegetables like kale, spinach, broccoli and cabbage.
- Introduce soy foods (e.g. soybeans, calcium-fortified soy milk, soy yogurt and tofu.) into daily eating.
- Eat regular amounts of fibre, especially soluble fibre.
- Stop eating fried foods.
- Don't consume potatoes regularly.
- Add regular helpings of beans and lentils.
- Choose extra virgin olive oil, canola, wheat germ and flaxseed oil.

Review Questions

1. What do you understand by endocrine system?
2. What are the types of diabetes? Explain them one by one.

3. Describe various symptoms of diabetes. How can we cure diabetes with food?
4. What are hyperthyroidism and hypothyroidism? Write down their dietary management.
5. Write a note on menopause and PCOD along with dietary management.

Disorders of Skeletal System

Arthritis

Arthritis is a term that includes a group of disorders that affect the joints and muscles. Arthritis symptoms include joint pain, inflammation and limited movement of joints. When a joint is inflamed it may be swollen, tender, warm to the touch or red. Surrounding each joint is a protective capsule holding a lubricating fluid to aid in motion. Cartilage, a slippery smooth substance, covers most joints to assure an even, fluid motion of the joint. With joint arthritis, the cartilage may be damaged, narrowed and lost by a degenerative process or by inflammation making movement painful.

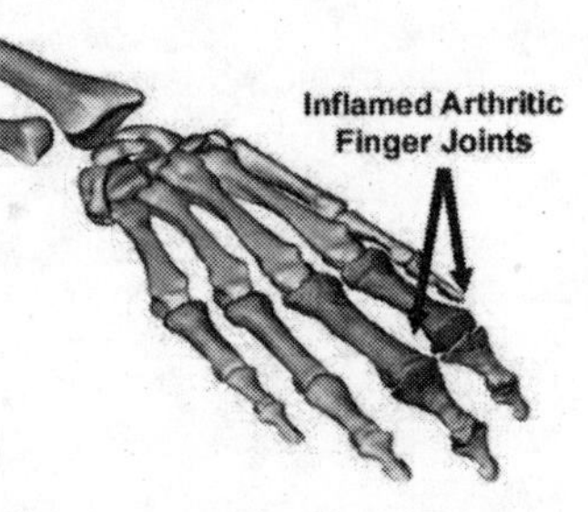

There are many different signs and symptoms of arthritis. These arthritis symptoms may come up suddenly or slowly over time and may also include sleeplessness, fatigue, depression and muscle aches. Many people experience some difficulty functioning at home, at work or at play because of joint pain, stiffness and loss of motion regardless of the type of arthritis they have. Getting out of bed in the morning, buttoning buttons, writing, sewing, meal preparation, dressing, sleeping, walking, climbing stairs, arising from a chair or a toilet seat and attending to matters of personal hygiene may all be impaired to some degree by arthritis pain and joint stiffness. A lot of people find that impairment of mobility is more distressing to them than arthritis pain.

Arthritis—Inflammation of a joint, marked by pain, heat, redness, and swelling. Arthritic disorders are among the most common chronic conditions that are painful and disabling. There are different types of arthritic disorders, most common include:

a) **Rheumatoid arthritis**

b) **Osteoarthritis**

c) **Septic arthritis**

d) **Gout**

Rheumatoid Arthritis

Rheumatoid arthritis or **RA**—This chronic, systemic inflammatory disease mainly attacks peripheral joints, surrounding muscles, tendons, ligaments, and blood vessels. Spontaneous remissions mark the course of rheumatoid arthritis. This disorder has the potential to cripple and in some cases patient becomes totally disable from severe articular deformity or associated extra articular symptoms, or both. In most patients, the disease follows an intermittent course and allows normal activity.

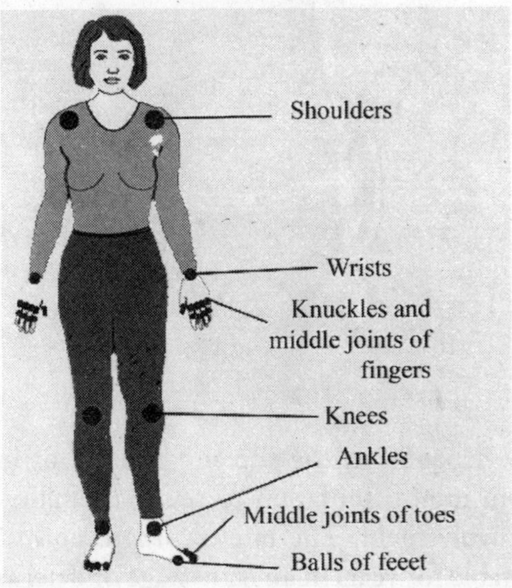

Joints frequently affected by Arthritis

Symptoms

Early stage—Fatigue, malaise, anorexia, persistent low-grade fever, and weight loss etc.

Later stage—Joint pain—joint symptoms occur bilaterally and symmetrically, tenderness, warmth and swelling, stiffness in hands and feet, weak, and painful muscles, May develop rheumatoid nodules (subcutaneous, round or oval, non tender masses, usually on pressure areas, such as the elbow)

Advance signs—Joint deformities and diminished joint function

Osteoarthritis

Osteoarthritis—The most common form of arthritis, this chronic condition causes deterioration of the joint cartilage and formation of reactive new bone at the margins and subchondral areas of the joints. Degeneration results from a breakdown of chondrocytes, most often in the hips and knees.

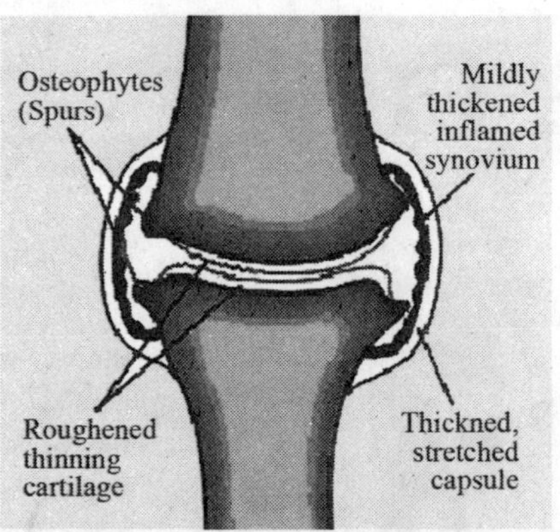

Disability depends on the site and severity of involvement and can range from minor limitation to severe disability in people with hip or knee involvement. The rate of progression varies, and joints may remain stable for years in an early stage of deterioration. Primary osteoarthritis, a normal part of aging, results from various things, such as metabolic, genetic, chemical, and mechanical factors. Secondary osteoarthritis usually follows an identifiable predisposing event, most commonly trauma or congenital deformity, which may lead to degenerative changes.

Symptoms

Signs and symptoms increase with poor posture, obesity, and occupational stress. Joint pain—that occurs particularly after exercise or weight bearing and that is usually relieved by rest. Stiffness in the morning and after exercise that is usually relieved by rest, aching during changes in weather, 'Grating' of the joint during motion and limited movement.

Septic Arthritis

It is a medial emergency. Bacteria invade a joint, resulting in inflammation of the synovial lining and leads to eventual destruction of bone and cartilage.

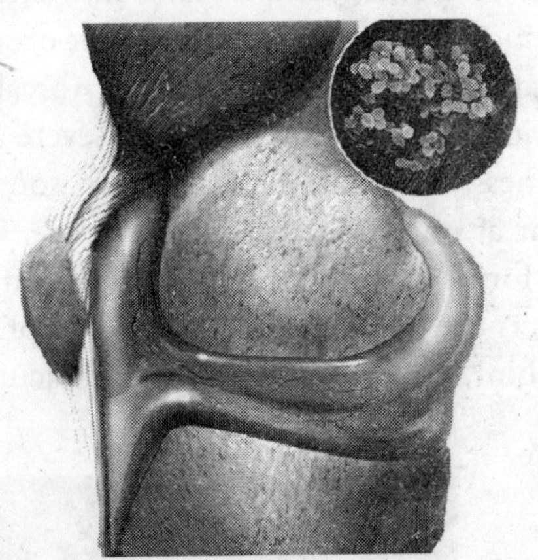

Septic

Causes—In most cases, bacteria spread from a primary site of infection, usually in adjacent bone or soft tissue, through the bloodstream to the joint.

There are various factors that can predispose a person to septic arthritis. Any concurrent bacterial infection or serious chronic illness (such as renal failure, diabetes, or cirrhosis) heightens susceptibility. Intravenous drug abuse can also cause septic arthritis. Other predisposing factors include recent articular trauma, joint surgery, intra articular injections, and local joint abnormalities.

Symptoms

Acute septic arthritis begins abruptly, causing intense pain, inflammation, and swelling of the affected joint, with low-grade fever. Most often develops in the large joints but can strike any joint, including the spine and small peripheral joints. Systemic signs of inflammation may not appear in some patients. If the bacteria invade the hip, pain may occur in the groin, upper thigh, or buttock.

Gout

Gout has been known for centuries. It can affect men of any age. It is less common in women and occurs only after the menopause. Gout is a systemic disease (i.e. condition that occurs throughout the body) caused by the buildup of uric acid (breakdown product of protein) in the joints. Gout causes sudden severe attacks of pain and tenderness, redness, warmth and swelling in some joints. It usually affects one joint at one time, often the big toe. Gout is one of the most common forms of arthritis or inflammation of a joint. It most commonly affects the big toe joints (Metatorsophalangeal joint) but can affect any joint. Gout usually starts as an acute attack that often

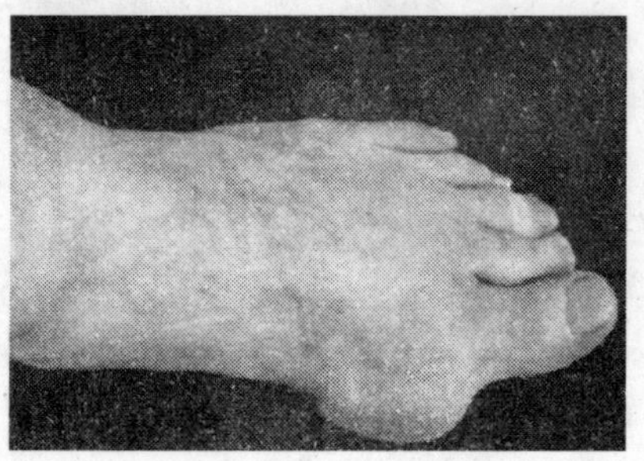

comes on overnight. With in 12 to 24 hours there is usually severe pain and swelling in the joint.

Types of Gout

There are three main types of "Gout":

a) **True "gout"**, which is the result of overly high uric acid naturally occurring in the system.

b) **"Pseudo-gout"**, has nothing to do with "gout" as such, but is a symptomatically gout-like condition involving calcium deposits on the bones of the foot.

c) **"Secondary Gout"**, which is gout condition arising from high uric acid in the blood, but caused by a drug used for another medical purpose. Hence the name "secondary".

> The normal amount of uric acid in the blood or serum depends on the person's gender. Males can have levels of 3.5 to 7.2 mg/dL (milligrams per deciliter), but females should only have 2.6 to 6.0 mg/dL.

Symptoms

Episodes develop very quickly and the first episode often occurs at night. These attacks may be caused by drinking too much alcohol, eating too much of certain foods, surgery, sudden serious illness, crash diets, joint injuries and chemotherapy. If there is no treatment the gout attack usually subsides in a week or so, after the first attack there may be intervals of many months or even years before there are other attacks. Overtime these attacks tend to become more frequent and more severe and eventually may involve other joints. Without treatment the state of chronic or continuous joint symptoms may develop with progressive joints damage. Gout generally occurs in four (4) stages (asymptomatic, acute, intercritical and chronic) and has the following signs and symptoms:

a) **Asymptomatic Stage**—urate levels rise in the blood, but produces no symptoms

b) **Acute Stage**—symptoms usually last from five to ten days

- Sudden attack of joint pain
- Swelling
- Joints feel hot, tender and look dusty red or bruised

c) **Intercritical Stage**—symptom-free intervals between gout episodes. Most people have a second attack from six months to two years, while others are symptom-free for five to 10 years.

d) **Chronic Stage**

- Persistently painful joints with large urate deposits in the cartilage, membranes between the bones, tendons and soft tissues.
- Skin over the deposits develop sores and release a white pus
- Joint stiffness
- Limited motion of the affected joint

Causes

Uric acid is the culprit. Gout results from a build up of too much uric acid in the body. High levels (High blood uric acid is defined as a serum urate level more than 7 mg/100 mL for adult males and 6 mg/100 mL for adult females) will cause crystals to form in cooler parts of the body (hence the toes and feet). Once these crystals form, the body's immune system thinks they are the foreign substances and attacks them. This causes the pain and swelling .The joints are not the only part of the body to be affected. Crystals may appear under the skin, usually sometimes on ears. They look like little white pimples and are called tophi. Gout can be inherited or may happen as a complication of another condition. Gout runs in families. The cause of gout is related to physiology of uric acid, which is a chemical that is the natural part of the common breaking down and building up of food and body tissues. Uric acid normally forms when the body breaks down the purines. When uric acid levels are higher, the condition is known as hyperuricemia. Uric acid is normally dissolved in blood but when it is high microscopic crystals may be deposited in the joint. As a result of this physiology gout is common in those, with hyperuricemia.

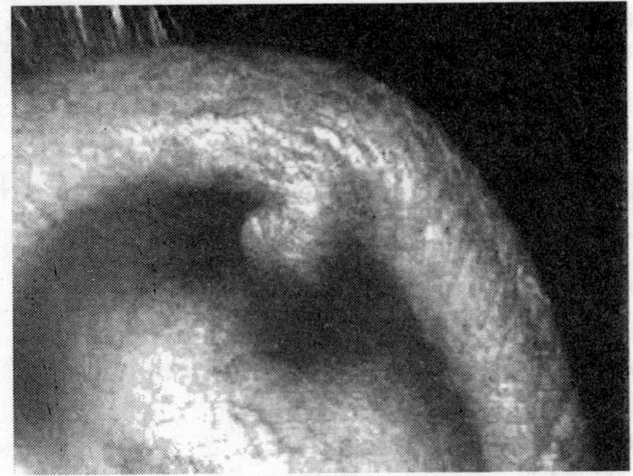

Tophi

Other causes of Gout include:

1. Some people just have higher levels and its hereditary
2. Obesity
3. High alcohol intake
4. High intake of foods that contain purines
5. Some of the drugs used to treat high blood pressure can lead to a gouty attack. Those with kidney disease may also develop high levels of uric acid.

Diagnosis

1. Physical examination and medical history
2. Blood test to measure uric acid
3. Joint fluid test to test for presence of uric acid crystals

Risk Factors

Approximately 18 percent of people who develop gout have a family history of the condition. Disease and conditions that increase the risk include diabetes, obesity, kidney disease and sickle cell anemia, regularly drinking alcohol interferes with the removal of uric acid from the body and can increase the risk of developing gout. Other risk factors include exposure to lead in the environment, high dietary intake of rich foods that contain purine. Medications that interfere with the body's ability to remove uric acid.

Signs

Inflammation, pain, redness, stiffness and swelling.

Gout Complications

Repeated attacks of gout may damage joints and cause arthritis.

Dietary Management

The following objectives should always be kept in mind:–

1. To control the uric acid levels in the blood.
2. To control and maintain IBW (ideal body weight).
3. To provide relief from symptoms.
4. To maintain optimal nutrition status.

A protein and calorie restricted diet has to be followed to lower the uric acid levels in the blood. To achieve the above objectives the following modifications in the diet are required.

Energy—The energy requirements have to be curtailed in case of the overweight individuals as losing weight lowers the uric acid levels in the blood.

Protein—Protein content of the diet has to be reduced, as uric acid is a breakdown product of protein.

Fat—Fat content of the diet has to be restricted especially oils that have been subjected to heat as in case of fried foods.

Fluids—Consume plenty of water. Fluid intake promotes the excretion of uric acid.

List of Foods

Foods recommended	Foods restricted	Foods to be avoided
Chapattis, rice and other cereals, cucumber, salads (without dressings), Fresh fruits.	Fats and oils to be restricted to 5-6 tsp/ day, Pulses.	Lentils, sweet bread, buns, peas, mushrooms, spinach, tomato, cauliflower, asparagus. Any kind of meats especially organ meats, dry fruits, nuts and peanuts. Fatty foods like cakes and pies leave the sugar products, excess of lemon juice, vinegar, and pickle, diuretics like alcohol, caffeine, tea and coffee.

Yeast and Uric Acid

The yeast used by brewers and bakers is called Saccharomyces cerevisiae, which uses sugar to produce carbon dioxide and alcohol. Flavoursome compounds are also produced. This single-cell fungus is rich in nutrients, especially water-soluble vitamins, like thiamin and folic acid, and some trace elements, like zinc and copper. The yeast contributes to the nutritional quality of a product like bread or beer. Alone, yeast is nothing but cells and their nuclei. This means that the relative concentration of material from the nuclei, like nucleic acid and purines, is high. As a consequence yeast increases the production of uric acid, after it has been eaten. This usually does not matter, since the body's capacity to handle it is adequate. Moreover, the associated alcohol in beer, for example, causes relatively more uric acid production in the body than would the nucleic acid from yeast.

Prevention

Prevention is the best defense against gout. Medications for example (small doses of non steroidal inflammatory drugs) may prevent continued accumulation of uric acid in the joints and further attack.

Other preventive measure may include the following:

- Drink at least 6-8 eight glasses of water, fresh juices or herb tea daily, especially at the first signs of gout. This will keep the urine diluted and will help body excrete uric acid and prevent crystals from forming.
- Eat foods high in potassium.
- Exercise regularly.
- Eating generous amounts of other fruits and vegetables help in keeping uric acid crystals in solution.
- Flavonoid containing foods should be part of the permanent gout-prevention diet.
- Having sex prevents men from getting gout. It seems that increased sexual activity reduces uric acid levels in fertile men.
- Lemon juice prevents gout attacks by stimulating the formation of calcium carbonate in the body. Calcium carbonate neutralizes acids in the body, including uric acid that triggers gout attacks. After each meal drink the juice of one freshly squeezed lemon in a glass of lukewarm water. But excess of lemon should be avoided.
- Taking ½ teaspoon of baking soda with meals will prevent gout attacks. This will help alkalize the body.
- A high fiber diet also helps in the elimination of uric acid by absorbing bile acids formed in the liver. These bile acids can act as a precursor to uric acid.

Low Purine Content Foods—Allowed (below 50mg purine per 100 gms of edible portion)

1. Milk and milk products
2. Eggs
3. Cereals
4. Vegetables except those listed below
5. Fruits
6. Sugar and sweets (must be restricted if the person is obese)
7. Fats and oils (1–2 tbsp. per day)
8. Nuts

Restricted Purine Content Foods (50–500 mg purine per 100 gms of edible portion)

1. Pulses 1 cup per day but exclude during an acute attack
2. Vegetables like peas, beans, spinach, apple, mushrooms and cauliflower

Avoided—High Purine Content Foods (500–1000 mg purine per 100 gms of edible portion)

1. Meat
2. Fish especially white bait, sardines, and herring.
3. Liver
4. Kidney
5. Heart
6. Pancreas
7. Sweet bread
8. Crab
9. Brain

Review Questions

1. What is arthritis? Write down the various arthritic disorders.
2. What is gout? Discuss its symptoms.
3. Write down the dietary management of gout.
4. What are purines? Enlist various low purine foods.
5. What is uric acid? What is its normal level in the blood?

Weight Management

Weight management means keeping body weight at a healthy level. Healthy weight management depends on sensible goals and expectations. Regular exercise and a healthy diet are must when it comes to controlling weight. A weight management plan depends on whether an individual is overweight or underweight.

Obesity and Overweight

Obesity is a complex, multifactorial condition in which excess body fat may put a person at health risk. Excess body fat results from an imbalance of energy intake and energy expenditure (total energy expenditure includes energy expended at rest, in physical activity and for metabolism). Obesity is considered a long-term complex disease. When the weight of a person is 20 percent more than his ideal body weight, he is said to be obese and when 10 percent more, then he is overweight.

Obese—A person who is 20 percent more than the normal ideal body weight for his sex, age and height.

Overweight—A person whose weight is 10 to 20 percent more than the normal ideal weight for his sex, age and height.

Fat is a normal component of the human body that is stored in adipose tissue. Obesity can be defined as a condition of excessive fat accumulation to the extent that health and well-being are affected. The fat may be equally distributed on the body, on the stomach (**apple-shaped**) or on the hips and thighs (**pear-shaped**).

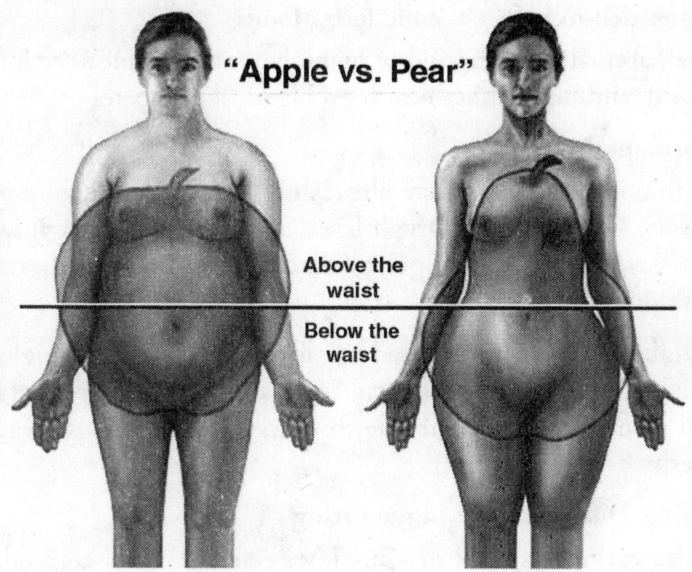

Causes

Being obese or overweight is generally caused by the intake of more calories than are expended by the body. Factors responsible for this are as follows:

- **Limited exercise and sedentary lifestyle**

  Sedentary lifestyle is one of the principal causes for obesity as physical activity is one of the greatest factors of the use of body energy. The increase in physical activity allows the intake of more calories and achieves a more favorable caloric balance of the body to avoid obesity.

- **Overeating**

  Intake of more calories than the body actually requires definitely causes the calories to accumulate in the body and for every 7,500 calories, the body gains 1kg of fat, which leads to obesity.

- **Inherited**

  Obesity tends to run in the families, suggesting a genetic cause.

- **A diet rich in high glycemic index foods**

  The habitual consumption of high-glycemic load meals results in obesity and many other health problems like diabetes.

- **Hormone Imbalances**

  Hormone imbalances may also cause obesity. Few examples of this are Cushing Illness (high levels of cortisol), hypothyroidism (low levels of thyroids), polycystic ovary syndrome and growth hormone deficiency etc.

- **Metabolic Disorders**, caused by the attempts to lose weight by weight cycling (also known as Yo-yo dieting, is a repeated loss and gain of body weight due to excessive dieting) also lead to obesity.

- **Eating Disorders like binge eating**

  Binge eating disorder is sometimes referred to as compulsive overeating. Binge eating disorder is more common in people who are obese or overweight, but it affects people with healthy weights as well. Binge eating and compulsive overeating are often termed as "addiction to food" because people who suffer from this disorder eat large amounts of food in very short periods of time. These overeating episodes are called "binges," and this causes obesity.

- **Stress**

  It has been estimated that about 80 percent of all illnesses and health problems are directly or indirectly related to stress, obesity is just one of them. Stress causes increased pituitary secretion of ACTH (adrenocorticotropic hormone) that results in an elevation of cortisol and a shift in fat distribution to the abdomen. Chronically stressed people with high cortisol levels develop a corresponding increase in abdominal fat deposits.

- **Insufficient and Irregular Sleep**

  Recent studies suggest that short sleep duration is independently associated with obesity in the general population.

- **Eating Too Many High-Fat or Refined Sugary Foods**

  The type of food eaten also plays an important role in the onset of obesity. The refined foods are known to interfere with food and energy metabolism in the body, and cause excessive fat storage.

- **Family Influences**

  Family diet and lifestyle are important contributory causes to modern child obesity. Parental behavioural patterns concerning shopping, cooking, eating and exercise, have an important influence on a child's energy balance and ultimately their weight. This is the reason why obese children and adolescents frequently grow up to be obese adults, it's clear that family influence also extends to adult obesity.

- **Metabolic**

  Some people are born with fast metabolisms. They burn fat easily. Others have slower metabolisms and burn fat slowly.

Ectomorph—The skinny person with a linear appearance, small muscles, low body fat, narrow shoulders, hips, waist and with an ultra fast metabolism.

Endomorph—The naturally large person characterised by a round face, wide hips, big bones, soft and plump body with slow metabolism and high number of fat cells.

Mesomorph—The naturally muscular person with wide shoulders, small waist, athletic build, low body fat percentage with an increased metabolism. Such a person tends to be active.

Complications of Obesity

There are many diseases, which are caused because of the obesity:

- Cholesterol, triglycerides and LDL cholesterol levels are co-related with obesity. All these increase the risk of heart ailments and hypertension.
- Uric acid levels also show similar relationship suggesting that obesity increases the risk of arthritic disorders like gout.

- Cortisol production is increased both in men and women while the testosterone levels decrease in men.
- Mechanical Disabilities like flat feet, respiratory problems, osteoarthritis, and varicose veins etc.
- Most of the diseases like coronary artery disease, hypertension, diabetes, gallstones, hernia, arthritis, gout, varicose veins, respiratory distress and even accidents are consequence of obesity and increase the risk of mortality.

Besides the medical problems the social complications are more immediate and may be very painful. The problem may start at school, affects the job opportunities and social status.

Measurement of Obesity

The degree to which a person is overweight or obese is generally described using an indication of the amount of excess body fat present. There are several common ways to measure the amount of fat present in an individual's body.

- **Simple Weighing**—This is the easiest and most common method, but by far the least accurate, as it only measures weight and does not take into account height, body type, and amount of muscle mass etc. The weight of the individual is measured and compared to an estimated ideal weight.
- **Body Mass Index(BMI)**—Body mass index assesses the body weight relative to height. It's a useful, indirect measure of body composition because it correlates highly with body fat. Weight in kilograms is divided by height in meters squared (kg/m^2). This is an adaptation of simple weighing which attempts to take into account the subject's general body size by dividing the weight by the height squared. This provides a slightly more accurate representation than simply measuring raw weight, but still ignores many factors which can affect the results, and is generally not accurate for many individuals.
- BMI values less than 18.5 are considered underweight.

- BMI values from 18.5 to 24.9 are healthy.
- Overweight is defined as a body mass index of 25.0 to less than 30.0 (grade I).
- Obesity is defined as a BMI of 30.0 or greater. People with BMI's of 30 or more are at higher risk of cardiovascular disease (grade II).
- Extreme obesity is defined as a BMI of 40 or greater (grade III).
- **Skinfold test**—With this method, the skin at several specific points on the body is pinched and the thickness of the resulting fold is measured. This measures the thickness of the layers of fat located under the skin, from which a general measurement of total amount of fat in the body is calculated. This method can be reasonably accurate for many people, but it does assume particular patterns for fat distribution over the body which may not apply to all individuals, and does not account for fat deposits which may not be directly under the skin. Also, as the measurement and analysis generally involves a high degree of practice and interpretation, for an accurate result it must be performed by a professional and cannot generally be done by patients themselves.

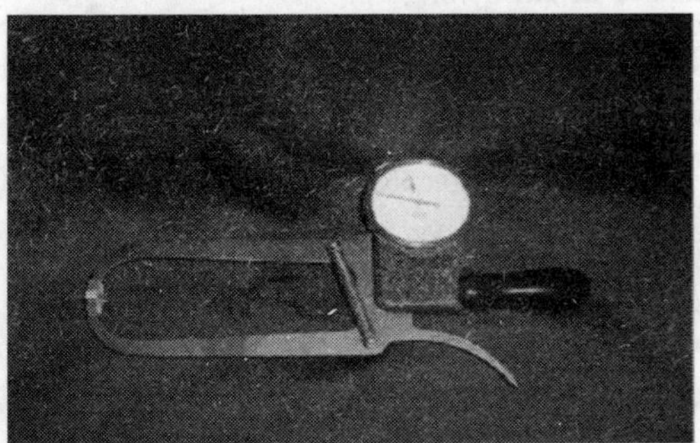

Calliper used for skinfold test

Treatment of Obesity

- Eat a low calorie or carbohydrate diet (Negative calorie balance).
- Small frequent meals.

- A high fibre and a low fat diet.
- Regular exercise improves the fitness of obese people and their feeling of well-being.

Weight Management and Energy Balance

Basal Metabolic Rate–BMR

Basal metabolic rate, or **BMR**, is the minimum calorific requirement needed to sustain life in a resting individual. This is the amount of energy, the body would burn if an individual sleeps the whole day (24 hours).

BMR is responsible for burning up to 60 to 70 percent of the total calories expended, but this figure varies depending upon different factors. Calories are needed for various bodily processes such as heart beating, inhaling and exhaling air, digesting food, making new blood cells, maintaining body temperature and every other metabolic process in the body.

BMR is the largest factor in determining overall metabolic rate and how many calories one needs to maintain, lose or gain weight. BMR is determined by a combination of genetic and environmental factors, which are as follows:

- **Genetics**—Some people are born with faster metabolisms, some with slower metabolisms.
- **Gender**—Men have a greater muscle mass and a lower body fat percentage. So they have a higher basal metabolic rate than women.
- **Age**—BMR decreases with age. After 20 years, it drops about 2 per cent every ten years.
- **Weight**—Heavier the weight, higher the BMR e.g. the metabolic rate of obese women is 25 percent higher than the metabolic rate of thin women.
- **Body Surface Area**—This is a reflection of the height and weight. The greater the body surface area factor, the higher the BMR. Tall, thin people have higher BMR.

- **Body Fat Percentage**—The lower the body fat percentage, the higher the BMR. The lower body fat percentage in the male body is one reason why men generally have a 10-15 percent faster BMR than women.

- **Diet**—Starvation or serious abrupt calorie reduction can dramatically reduce BMR by up to 30 percent. Restrictive low-calorie weight loss diets may cause the BMR to drop as much as 20 percent.

- **Body Temperature and Health**—For every increase of 1°F in internal temperature of the body, the BMR increases by about 7 percent. The chemical reactions in the body actually occur more quickly at higher temperatures.

- **External Temperature**—Temperature outside the body also affects basal metabolic rate. Exposure to cold temperature causes an increase in the BMR, so as to create the extra heat needed to maintain the body's internal temperature. A short exposure to hot temperature has little effect on the body's metabolism as it is compensated mainly by increased heat loss. But prolonged exposure to heat can raise BMR.

- **Glands**—Thyroxin (produced by the thyroid gland) is a key BMR-regulator which speeds up the metabolic activity of the body. The more thyroxin produced, the higher the BMR. If too much thyroxin is produced (a condition known as thyrotoxicosis) BMR can actually double. If too little thyroxin is produced (myxoedema) BMR may shrink to 30 to 40 percent of the normal. Like thyroxin, adrenaline also increases the BMR but to a lesser extent.

- **Exercise**—Physical exercise not only influences body weight by burning calories but it also helps raise the BMR by building extra lean tissue.

- **Malnutrition**—Malnutrition lowers the BMR.

Lean tissue (muscle), is more metabolically demanding than fat tissue. It requires a great deal of energy just to sustain it. It is obvious then that one way to increase the BMR is to engage in weight training in order to increase or maintain lean body mass. In this manner it could be said that weight training helps lose body fat indirectly.

Short Term Factors, which affect BMR

- Illnesses such as a fever.
- High levels of stress hormones in the body.
- Either an increase or decrease in the environmental temperature will result in an increase in BMR.
- Fasting, starving or malnutrition, which results in the lowering of BMR.

Calculation of Total daily energy expenditure (TDEE)

Total daily energy expenditure (TDEE) is the total number of calories that the body expends in 24 hours, including all activities. TDEE is also known as the "maintenance level". Caloric expenditure can vary widely and is much higher for athletes or extremely active individuals. Calorie requirements may also vary among otherwise identical individuals due to differences in inherited metabolic rates.

There are many different formulas of determining the caloric maintenance level by taking into account the factors of age, sex, height, weight, lean body mass, and activity level. Any formula that takes into account the lean body mass (LBM) gives the most accurate determination of the energy expenditure. A much more accurate method for calculating TDEE is to determine basal metabolic rate (BMR) using multiple factors, including height, weight, age and sex, then multiply the BMR by an activity factor to determine TDEE.

TDEE = Activity factor x BMR

The Harris-Benedict formula for calculating BMR based on total body weight

The Harris Benedict equation formula uses the factors of height, weight, age, and sex to determine basal metabolic rate (BMR). This makes it more accurate than determining calorie needs based on total body weight alone. The only variable it does not take into consideration is lean body mass. Therefore, this equation will be very accurate in all but not in the extremely muscular and the extremely overfat people.

Men: BMR = 66 + (13.7 x wt in kg) + (5 X ht in cm)–(6.8 x age in years)

Women: BMR = 655 + (9.6 x wt in kg) + (1.8 x ht in cm)–(4.7 x age in years)

Note: 1 inch = 2.54 cm.

1 kilogram = 2.2 lbs.

Katch-McArdle formula for calculating BMR based on lean body weight

This formula from Katch and McArdle takes into account lean mass and therefore is more accurate than a formula based on total body weight. The Harris Benedict equation has separate formulas for men and women because men generally have a higher LBM and this is factored into the men's formula. Since the Katch-McArdle formula accounts for LBM, this single formula applies equally to both men and women. For using Katch-McArdle formula one must get body composition tested.

BMR (men and women) = 370 + (21.6 X lean mass in kg)

Example:

Calculate BMR for a female whose weight is 54.5 kg, body fat percentage is 20 percent (24 lbs. fat) and lean mass is 43.6 kg.

BMR = 370 + (21.6 X 43.6) = 1312 calories

Activity Multiplier

Sedentary = BMR x 1.2 (little or no exercise, desk job)

Lightly active = BMR x 1.375 (light exercise/sports 1–3 days/wk)

Moderately active = BMR x 1.55 (moderate exercise/sports 3–5 days/wk)

Very active = BMR x 1.725 (hard exercise/sports 6–7 days/wk)

Extremely active = BMR x 1.9 (hard daily exercise/sports and physical job)

Example

Calculate the Total daily energy expenditure (TDEE) of a moderately active woman whose BMR is 1245 kcal per day.

BMR is 1245 kcal per day

Activity level is moderately active so the activity factor is 1.55

TDEE = 1.55 x 1245 = 1929.75 calories/day

Negative calorie balance for obese and overweight patients

Weight gain is caused when the calorie intake exceeds the calorie expenditure. If calorie expenditure exceeds the calorie intake negative calorie balance occurs which leads to weight loss. Some foods get stored as fat more easily than others, but too much of anything, even "healthy food," gets stored as fat. One must be in a calorie deficit to burn fat. This forces the body to use stored body fat to make up for the energy deficit. There are 3500 calories in a pound of stored body fat. If an individual creates a 3500-calorie deficit in a week through diet, exercise or a combination of both, he or she can lose one pound. The calorie deficit can be created through diet, exercise or preferably, with a combination of both. It should always be kept in mind that cutting calories in excess slows down the metabolic rate, decreases thyroid output and causes loss of lean mass. The most common guideline for calorie deficits for fat loss is to reduce the calories by at least 500, but not more than 1000 below the maintenance level. For some, especially lighter people, 1000 calories may be too much of a deficit. A more individualized way to determine the safe calorie deficit would be to account for one's bodyweight or TDEE.

Reducing calories by 15–20 percent below TDEE is a good place to start. A larger deficit may be necessary in some cases, but the best approach would be to keep the calorie deficit through diet small while increasing activity level.

Example—If a person weighs 55 kg, TDEE is 2033 calories, calorie deficit to lose weight is 500 calories then optimal caloric intake for weight loss is 2033–500 = 1533 calories.

Or

Calorie deficit to lose weight is 20 percent of TDEE (0.20 x 2033 = 406 calories) the optimal caloric intake for weight loss = 2033–406= **1627 calories**

Bulimia Nervosa

Bulimia nervosa, often abbreviated to bulimia, is an eating disorder where people have a cycle of binge-eating and purging. People with bulimia have an intense dread of putting on weight. Bulimia is most common in teenage girls and young women, although anyone can develop the illness at any age.

Underweight

Underweight is a condition in which the person does not have an ideal body weight as per his height and sex. The person usually weighs about 10 percent below the ideal weight. Sometimes, the problem of underweight is hereditary. But, there are other factors like metabolic disorders that can be responsible for causing underweight. The definition is usually made with reference to the body mass index (BMI). Most individuals under BMI 18.5 are considered to be underweight. But as BMI is a statistical estimate, some individuals classified as underweight may be perfectly healthy.

Underweight—A person who is 10 percent or more below the normal ideal body weight for his sex, age and height.

Causes

The most common cause of underweight is malnutrition which is caused by the unavailability of adequate food. There are many causes of underweight, which are as follows:

- Inadequate nutrition or bad eating habits
- Cancer
- Tuberculosis
- Anorexia nervosa and bulimia
- Hyperthyroidism
- Diabetes (especially type 1)
- Anxiety and depressive disorders
- Diseases of digestive system
- Feebleness, especially in the elderly
- Overtraining
- HIV/AIDS
- Drug abuse
- Decreased fat forming tendency of the body
- Infections
- Malabsorption syndromes
- Hormone Disorders

Treatment of Underweight

The individuals who are severely underweight usually suffer from other health problems as well. Such patients really need to gain weight. The treatment for an underweight individual is to increase the calorie intake. Exercises which increase the muscle mass should be continued.

Positive calorie balance to gain body weight

If an individual wants to gain body weight, he/she must consume more calories and should also participate in a weight-training program of a sufficient intensity, frequency and volume, the caloric surplus will be used to create new muscle tissue. Once determining the total daily energy expenditure (TDEE), the next step is to increase the calories high enough above TDEE that one can gain weight. It is a basic law of energy balance that one must be on a positive calorie balance diet to gain muscular body weight. A general guideline for a starting point for gaining weight is to add approximately 300–500 calories per day into TDEE. An alternate method is to add an additional 15 to 20 percent onto the TDEE.

Example—If a person weighs 55 kg, TDEE is 2033 calories, increased calorie intake to gain weight is 500 calories then optimal caloric intake for weight gain is 2033 + 500 = 2533 calories. Or the additional calorie requirement for weight gain is 15 to 20 percent i.e. 305–406 calories which means that optimal caloric intake for weight gain is 2033 + (305 to 406) = 2338–2439 calories.

Gradual adjustment of caloric intake

After calculating the total daily energy expenditure and adjusting it according to the goal, if the amount is substantially higher or lower than the current intake, then one may need to adjust the calories gradually. For example, if an individual caloric intake is 1900 calories per day, but he has only been eating 900 calories per day. Then his metabolism may be sluggish. An immediate jump to 1900 calories per day might actually cause a fat gain because the body has adapted to a lower caloric intake and the sudden jump up would create a surplus. The best approach would be to gradually increase the calories from 900 to 1900 over a period of a few weeks to allow the metabolism to speed up and acclimatize.

Adjustment of caloric intake according to the need (weight loss/ weight gain)

After calculating the TDEE (maintenance level), the next step is to adjust the calories according to the need. Following things should be kept in mind:

- To keep the weight at its current level, one should remain at the daily caloric maintenance level.
- To lose weight, one needs to create a calorie deficit by reducing the calories slightly below the maintenance level (or keeping the calories the same and increasing the activity above current level.
- To gain weight one need to increase the calories above maintenance level.

The only difference between weight gain programs and weight loss programs is the total number of calories required.

Body Shapes

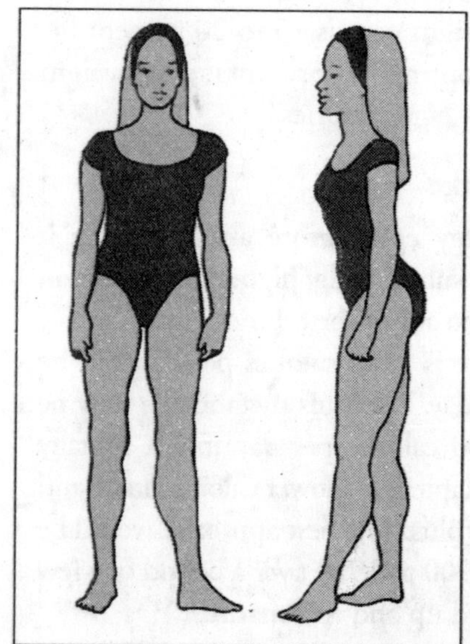

Ideal Android Body Shape

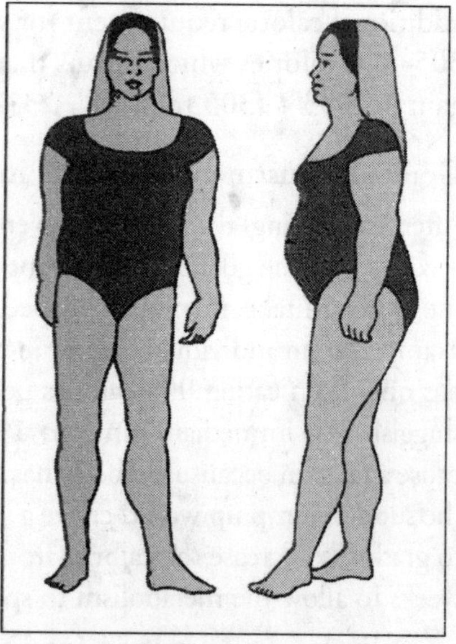

Overwight Android Body Shape

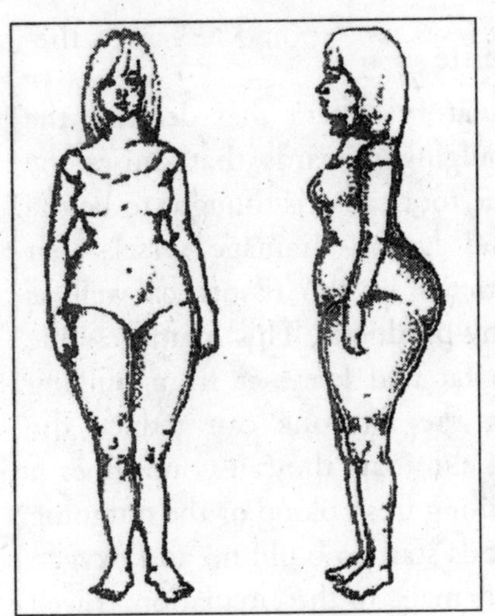

Overweight Gynaeoid Body Shape

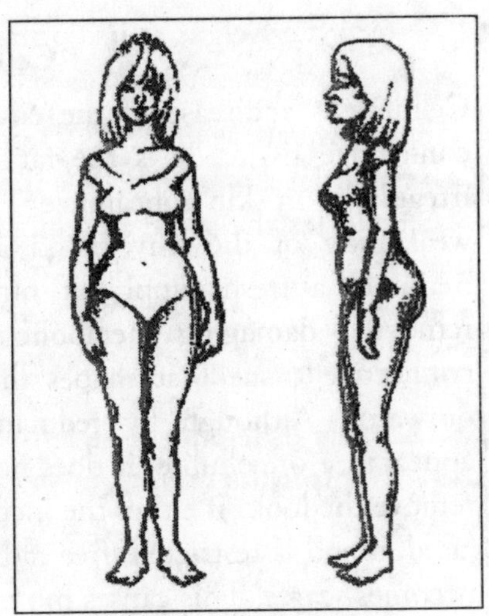

Ideal Gynaeoid Body Shape

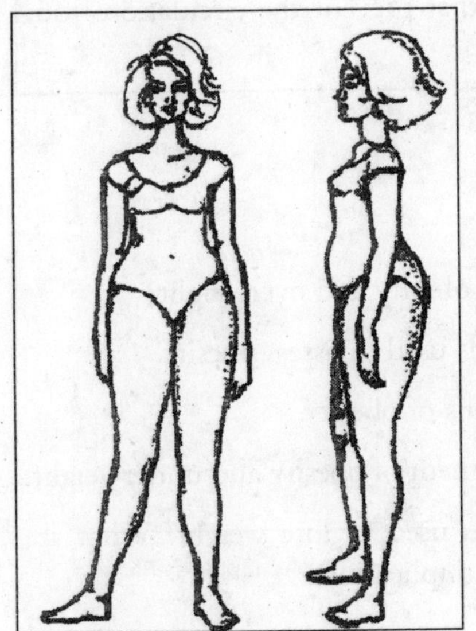

Overweight Thyroid Body Shape

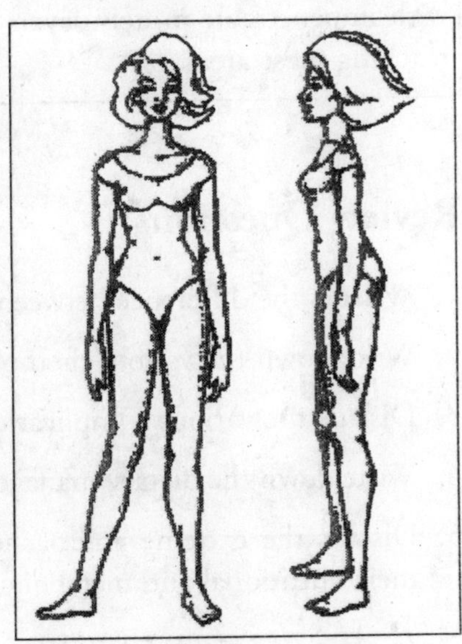

Ideal Thyroid Body Shape

Cellulite

Cellulite is a disease of the circulatory system that deforms the connective tissue. It is the fat bulging upwards that causes the irregularity in skin appearance. The root cause is thought to be the weakening of the tiny blood and lymph drainage vessels that maintain a fresh supply of nutrients in the tissues as well as removing damaging metabolic by-products. This damages the connective tissue that shapes the fat and keeps it from bulging outwards. Although by reducing the fat, one can reduce the appearance of cellulite, it does not eliminate the cause, nor does it remove the look. If either the incoming fresh blood or the outgoing 'used' blood is restricted, free radicals start to build up and oxygen becomes scarce. This causes more damage to the circulation as well as impairing the function of the cells that manage the structure of the connective tissue. These cells are known as fibroblasts and when they malfunction they cause two problems, they weaken of the fibers that hold the fat cells in place and they coat clumps of fat cells with impenetrable protein layers that prevent the circulation from reaching these areas.

Review Questions

1. What is the difference between obesity and overweight?
2. Write down the various methods used to assess obesity.
3. Discuss the various complications of obesity.
4. Write down the dietary management of obesity and underweight.
5. Discuss the extreme approaches used to lose weight. What are their nutritional and metabolic implications?

Home Remedies for Various Diseases

Acidity

- Eat a cup of vanilla ice cream or drink a glass of cold milk to get heartburn and acidity relief within minutes.
- Take a mixture of two teaspoon of natural apple cider vinegar and 2 tsp raw honey in a glass of water before meals.
- Take one piece of clove and suck on it slowly. This will give relief from acidity and also help in reducing the risk of diseases arising out of acidity.
- Avoid fried foods, pickles, hot spicy foods, vinegar, and chocolate.
- Eat a cup of ice cream or drink a glass of cold milk to get heartburn and acidity relief within minutes.
- Drink tender coconut water 3 to 4 times a day.
- Bananas, watermelon and cucumber have protective action against the acidity and heart burn. Eating a banana daily will prevent such conditions.
- Avoid raw salad of vegetables like onion, cabbage, radish, and peppers.
- A piece of jaggery should be placed in the mouth and sucked till, acidity subsides.
- Eat 4 to 5 almonds, whenever heartburns start.

- Chew the food properly. Do not eat in a hurry.
- Keep a minimum time interval between meals, as this decreases production of gas.
- Maintaining an upright/sitting procedure is helpful, as it prevents acid reflux (re-entry of acid).
- Drink plenty of water, at least 8 glasses daily.
- Do not eat just before going to bed. Eat around 1 to 2 hours, before sleeping.
- Discontinue smoking and cut down on alcohol.

Anorexia

- Oranges are an extremely useful remedy for anorexia. They stimulate the flow of digestive juices, thereby improving digestion and increasing appetite. One or two oranges a day are advised.
- Boil 2–3 cloves of garlic in 1 cup of water. Strain, Add the juice of half a lime to this and drink 2 times a day, for a week.
- Sour grapes are another effective remedy for anorexia. The juice of these grapes should be used in kneading the flour before preparing chapattis. These chapattis should be eaten continuously for two to three weeks. This remedy helps tone up the stomach and improve the appetite.
- Make a paste of fresh ginger. Add a pinch of salt and a drop of lime juice to half a teaspoon of the paste. Eat this 2 times a day for 1 week.
- Apples are also useful in anorexia. They help in digestion by stimulating the flow of pepsin, a protein digesting enzyme, in the stomach.
- Garlic possesses a special property to stimulate the digestive tone of the system and improves appetite. Three or four cloves of raw garlic should be boiled in a cup of water. A soup prepared from this vegetable can be of immense help to a patient suffering from anorexia.

Arthritis

- Warm mustard oil, spread it over madar leaf (Indian) and foment the joint by spreading the leaf over the joint and keep it there for few hours for arthritis relief.
- The raw potato juice therapy is considered one of the most successful biological treatments for rheumatic and arthritic conditions. It has been used in folk medicine for centuries. The traditional method of preparing potato juice is to cut a medium-sized potato into thin slices, without peeling the skin, and place the slices overnight in a large glass filled with cold water. The water should be drunk in the morning on an empty stomach. Fresh juice can also be extracted from potatoes. A medium-sized potato should be diluted with a cup of water and taken in the morning.
- One tablespoon juice of fresh leaves of bathua, drink every day on an empty stomach for 2–3 months. Do not add anything to the juice and do not eat anything for 2 hours before and after.
- A teaspoon of black sesame seeds, soaked in a quarter cup of water and kept overnight, has been found to be effective in preventing frequent joint pains. The water in which the seeds are soaked should also be taken along with the seeds in the morning.
- On an empty stomach take 3–4 walnuts (akhrot) or 1 fresh coconut.
- Garlic is another effective remedy for arthritis. It contains an anti-inflammatory property, which accounts for its effectiveness in the treatment of this disease. Garlic may be taken raw or cooked according to individual preference.
- Lime has also been found beneficial as a home remedy for arthritis. The citric acid found in lime is a solvent of uric acid, which is the primary cause of some types of arthritis. The juice of one lime, diluted with water, may be taken once a day, preferably first thing in the morning.

- Warm coconut oil or mustard oil, mixed with two or three pieces of camphor should be massaged on stiff and aching joints. It increases blood supply, and reduces inflammation and stiffness with the gentle warmth produced while massaging.

Asthma

- A teaspoon of fresh ginger juice, mixed with a cup of fenugreek decoction and honey to taste, acts as an excellent expectorant in cases of asthma.
- Ten garlic cloves, boiled in 30 ml of milk, are good for early stages of asthma. Steaming ginger tea with two garlic cloves in it, can also help to keep the problem under control.
- Honey is one of the most common home remedy for asthma. If a jug of honey is held under the nose of an asthma patient and he inhales the air that comes into contact with it, he starts breathing easier and deeper. One to two teaspoonful of honey taken with water or milk provide relief. It thins out accumulated mucus and helps its elimination from the respiratory passages.
- Figs have proved very valuable in asthma. They give comfort to the patient by draining off the phlegm. Three or four dry figs should be cleaned thoroughly with warm water and soaked overnight and should be taken early in the morning, along with the water in which they were soaked.
- Lemon is another fruit found beneficial in the treatment of asthma. The juice of one lemon, diluted in a glass of water and taken with meals, brings good results.
- Amla with one tablespoon of honey forms an effective medicinal tonic for the treatment of this disease. It should be taken every morning. When fresh fruit is not available, dry gooseberry powder can be mixed with honey.

- A decoction of linseed is also considered useful in curing congestion in asthma and preventing recurrence of attacks.
- During the attack, mustard oil, mixed with a little camphor, should be massaged over the back of the chest. This will loosen up phlegm and ease breathing.
- One of the preventive measures to stop attacks of asthma is to drink water, which has been kept overnight in a copper vessel. This water, with traces of copper in it, is believed to change one's constitutional tendency to get respiratory problems.

Boils

- Garlic and onions have proved most effective among the several home remedies found beneficial in the treatment of boils. The juice of garlic or onion may be applied externally on boils to help ripen them, break them, and evacuate the pus. An equal quantity of the juices of these two vegetables can also be applied with beneficial results. Eating two to three pods of garlic during meals also brings good results.
- Bitter gourd is another effective home remedy for blood-filled boils. A glassful of fresh juice of this vegetable, mixed with a teaspoon of lime juice, should be taken, daily for a few months to treat this condition.
- One teaspoon of milk cream, mixed with half a teaspoon of vinegar, and a pinch of turmeric powder, makes an excellent poultice. It helps in ripening the blood boils and in the healing without allowing them to become septic.
- Cumin seeds are beneficial in the treatment of boils. The seeds should be ground in water and made into a paste. This paste can be applied to boils with beneficial results.
- The use of margosa leaves has proved effective in boils. They can be used as a poultice, decoction, or liniment with beneficial results. To make the decoction, 15 gm of margosa leaves should be boiled in 500 ml of water till it is reduced by one-third.

- Application of turmeric powder on boils speeds up the healing process. In the case of fresh boils, a few dry roots of turmeric are roasted, the ashes dissolved in a cupful of water, and then applied over the affected portion. This solution enables the boils to ripen and burst.

Cough

- Drink hot milk with honey at bedtime for cough relief.
- Grapes are one of the most effective home remedies for the treatment of a cough. Grapes tone up the lungs and act as an expectorant, relieving a simple cold and cough in a couple of days. A cup of grape juice mixed with a teaspoon of honey is advised for cough relief.
- Almonds are useful for dry coughs. Seven kernels should be soaked in water overnight and the brown skin removed. They should then be ground well to form a fine paste. A quantity of twenty grams each of butter and sugar should then be added to the paste. This paste should be taken in the morning and evening.
- The use of raw onion is valuable in a cough. This vegetable should be chopped fine and the juice extracted from it. One teaspoon of the juice should then be mixed with one teaspoon of honey and kept for four or five hours—it will make an excellent cough syrup and should be taken twice daily.
- The root of the turmeric plant is useful in a dry cough. The root should be roasted and powdered. Three gram dose of this should be taken twice daily, in the morning and evening.
- Raisins are also useful in a cough. A sauce can be prepared by grinding 100 gm of raisins with water. About 100 gm of sugar should be mixed with it and then heated. Twenty grams should be taken at bedtime daily.
- Aniseed is another effective remedy for a hard dry cough with difficult expectoration. It breaks up the mucus. A tea made from this spice should be taken.

- In the case of a severe cough, the patient should take orange juice and water.

Constipation

- Bale fruit is the best laxative of all fruits. It cleans and tones up the intestines and gives relief from constipation.
- Giving bran may relieve constipation in toddlers, infants and older children.
- Guava when eaten with seeds provides roughage to diet which gives relief from constipation.
- Add more fruits to the diet like prunes, pears, grapes, orange juice and papaya.
- Try one tablespoonful of corn syrup added to half cup of water to cure constipation.
- Another natural remedy for constipation is to add a little extra sugar or some honey in a glass of milk. Drink twice a day.

Diabetes

- Soak 1 teaspoon of fenugreek seeds in 1 cup of water at night. Drink the water in the morning on an empty stomach and eat the seeds. Very good for diabetes because it works like insulin.
- Boil the 5 leaves each of tulsi (Basil), neem, jamun, bel, with 4 seeds of pepper in a glass of water and drink two times a day (persons with high blood pressure should avoid it).
- Morning and evening walk for at least 45 minutes is most essential to control this disease.
- Eat one teaspoon of cinnamon daily.

- Take one small bitter gourd, remove the seeds and saturate in a cup of water. Drain and drink every morning.
- Wash and peel a green plantain, put the peel in a jar, cover with water and drink this water three times a day.
- Boil 13–16 mango leaves in one cup of water, saturate over night and filter in the morning. Drink every morning on an empty stomach.
- Consume garlic daily.

Gout

- The cherry, sweet or sour, is considered effective in treating gout. To start with, the patient should consume about fifteen to twenty five cherries a day. Thereafter, about ten cherries a day will keep the ailment under control. While fresh cherries are best, canned cherries can also be used occasionally.
- Raw vegetable juices are used for gout treatment. Carrot juice, in combination with the juices of beet and cucumber, is especially valuable.
- The juice of french beans has also proved effective in treating gout. About 150 ml of this juice should be taken daily by the patient suffering from this disease.
- Apples are excellent for curing gout. The malic acid contained in them is believed to neutralise the uric acid and afford relief to gout sufferers. The patient is advised to take one apple after each meal.
- Bananas have been found beneficial in the treatment of gout. A diet of bananas only for three or four days is advised for providing some relief from gout. A patient can take eight or nine bananas daily during this period and nothing else.

- Lime is also used for treating gout. Vitamin C is known to prevent and cure sore joints by strengthening the connective tissues of the body. The citric acid found in lime dissolves uric acid which is the primary cause of this disease. The juice of half a lime, squeezed into a glass of water, should be taken twice daily.

High Blood Pressure and Heart Diseases

- Asparagus is an excellent food for strengthening the heart. A good medicine for a weak or an enlarged heart is prepared by mixing the freshly extracted juice of this vegetable with honey, in the ratio of 2:1. A teaspoon of this medicine should be taken three times daily.
- To reduce the blood pressure, daily take plain aerated water two to three times a day.
- Fresh fruits in general are beneficial in treating the heart diseases. They tone up the heart. Grapes are especially effective in heart pain and palpitation of the heart, and the disease can be rapidly controlled if the patient adopts an exclusive diet of grapes for few days. Grape juice is particularly valuable when one is actually suffering from a heart attack.
- It is possible to even reverse the heart problems by not using oil or ghee at all, by taking only boiled vegetables, doing yogic exercises, and by living a tension free life.
- Vitamin C is also essential as it protects against spontaneous breaches in capillary walls which can lead to heart attacks. It also guards against high blood cholesterol. The stress of anger, fear, disappointment and similar emotions can raise blood fat and cholesterol levels immediately but this reaction to stress can do little harm if the diet is adequate in vitamin C and pantothenic acid.
- Daily intake of lemon and ghia juice (bottle gourd) keeps the heart strong and reduces the blood pressure.

- Remember all spices and dry fruits produce cardiovascular diseases.
- Daily intake of sprouted grams and moong makes the heart muscles strong.
- Indian gooseberry (amla) is considered an effective home remedy for heart disease. It tones up the functions of all the organs of the body, and builds up health by destroying the heterogeneous elements and renewing lost energy. When the fruit is in season, one medium-sized Indian gooseberry can be taken with a little salt daily, when not in season, dry pieces can be chewed.
- Pranayam, or deep breathing exercises three times a day, at least for 15 minutes each, immediately reduce the blood pressure.
- It is very essential to take a minimum of 8 hours sound sleep every day.
- Apples have heart-stimulating properties. Patients suffering from a weak heart will benefit greatly by making liberal use of this fruit and apple jam.
- Onions have been found valuable in heart diseases. They are useful in maintaining the blood cholesterol levels by oxidising excess cholesterol. One teaspoon of raw onion juice taken early first in the morning is beneficial in such cases.
- Honey has got marvellous properties to prevent all sorts of heart diseases. It improves the circulation. It is also effective in cardiac pain. One tablespoon daily after food is sufficient to prevent all sorts of heart troubles.
- The herb alfalfa in the form of juice has been found very helpful in most troubles related to the arteries and heart diseases. Only the leaves of the plant are used for this purpose, when they can be obtained fresh. The juice of fresh alfalfa is, however, too strong and potent to be taken by itself. It is best taken with carrot juice in equal quantities of 125 ml each, twice daily. In this combination, the individual benefits of each juice are intensified.

- Safflower oil has proved beneficial in lowering blood cholesterol. Hence it can be used liberally with persons suffering from cardiovascular disorders.
- Mix ½ onion juice and ½ honey. Take two tablespoons once a day for 1–2 weeks.
- Patients with heart disease should increase their intake of foods rich in vitamin E, as this vitamin is said to promote heart function by improving oxygenation of the cells. It also improves the circulation and muscle strength. Many whole meal products and green vegetables, particularly outer leaves of cabbage, are good sources of vitamin E.
- Eat a papaya on an empty stomach daily for a month. Do not eat anything after for about 2 hours.

Jaundice

- The green leaves of radish are another valuable remedy for jaundice. The leaves should be pounded and their juice is extracted. Half a litre of this juice should be taken daily by an adult patient. It induces a healthy appetite and proper evacuation of bowels, and this results in gradual decrease of the trouble. In most cases, complete cure can be ensured within eight or ten days.
- Tomatoes are valuable in jaundice. A glass of fresh tomato juice, mixed with a pinch of salt and pepper, taken early in the morning, is considered an effective remedy for this disease.
- The leaves of snake gourd have also been found useful in jaundice.
- The juice of green leaves of pigeon pea is useful in jaundice. The juice extracted form these leaves should be taken in doses of 40 to 60 ml daily.

- A mixture of almonds, dried dates and cardamoms is an effective remedy for jaundice. seven kernels of almonds, one dried date, and three small cardamoms should be soaked overnight in water. The outer coating of the almond kernels and the inner seeds of dried dates should be removed the next morning and the whole material should be rubbed into a fine paste. Then, fifty to sixty grams of sugar and an equal amount of butter should be mixed in it.
- Lemon is also beneficial in the treatment of jaundice. The patient should be given lemon juice mixed with water several times a day. This will protect the damaged liver cells.
- Barley water is another good remedy for this disease. One cup of barley should be boiled in three litres of water and simmered for three hours.
- Add two teaspoons of basil juice to 40 to 50 ml of radish juice, add little jaggery to it. Drink this juice twice or three times a day for a month for total relief.

Loose Motion/Dysentery

- Make a paste of dry pomegranate seeds and raisin with a little of salt in it. It is a most effective remedy.

Menopausal Disorders

- During menopause, lack of ovarian hormones can result in severe calcium deficiency. For this reason, a larger than usual intake of calcium may help greatly. Vitamin D is also essential for assimilation of calcium. Any woman experiencing disturbing symptoms at this time should supplement her daily diet with vitamin D, magnesium, and calcium daily, which can be supplied by one litre of milk.
- Beet juice has been found very useful in menopausal disorders. It should be taken in small quantities of 60 to 90 ml at a time, thrice a day.

- Carrot seeds are good for relieving menopausal tension. A teaspoon of the seeds should be boiled in a glass of cow's milk for about ten minutes and taken daily as medicine in the treatment of this condition.
- The use of liquorice is one of the most effective remedies for menopausal disorders. Liquorice contains the natural female hormone, estrogen, and can, to some degree, compensate for the diminished hormone. One teaspoon of the powder should be taken daily.

Oedema

- Mustard oil is an effective home remedy for oedema. Take some warm mustard oil and rub it on the affected areas. Soak 2 teaspoons of mustard seeds in water and apply the solution in the affected areas.
- Fresh juice of beets, carrot and cucumber in quantities of 100 ml each, are one of the finest cleansers of the gall-bladder. This combined juice has proved beneficial in the treatment of all disorders related to this organ, and should be taken twice daily.
- The pear is another excellent remedy for gall-bladder disorders. The fruit or its juice should be taken liberally by the patient with beneficial results. It has a special healing effect on all gall-bladder disorders, including gallstones.
- Dandelion has a beneficial effect on the gall bladder. About 125 ml each of the juices of dandelion and watercress should be taken twice daily. Combined with a vegetarian diet, without much sugar and starch, these juices help to make the gall-bladder normal.

Obesity (Fatness)

- Eat the food by chewing a single morsel at least 50 times, so that it turns into almost a liquid before swallowing it down. Very effectively it reduces the obesity.

- Don't take meals under tension.
- Stop taking chapatti/bread prepared with wheat only. It should be a mixture of whole grams flour and soybeans.
- Take half lemon in hot water daily empty stomach in the morning.

Osteoporosis

- Getting regular exercise, especially weight-bearing and muscle strengthening exercises.
- Getting adequate vitamin D, whether through diet, exposure to sunshine, or supplements.
- Consuming enough calcium.
- Consuming adequate vitamin K, found in green-leafy vegetables.
- There is evidence that drinking a lot of coffee—about four or more cups per day—can increase the risk of fracture. Caffeine tends to promote calcium excretion in urine.
- Getting too much protein can leach calcium from the bones. As the body digests protein, it releases acids into the bloodstream, which the body neutralizes by drawing calcium from the bones. Animal protein seems to cause more of this calcium leaching than vegetable protein does.
- Don't take more of vitamin A. Preformed vitamin A can promote fractures. Vitamin A in the form of beta-carotene does not increase one's fracture risk.

Piles

- Wash 2 to 3 dried figs very well and soak in a glass of cold water overnight. Have it in the morning. Similarly have figs in the evening that have been soaked in the morning. Have them for 2-3 weeks for good results. It is effective treatment for ordinary piles as well as bleeding piles.

- Mix one teaspoon fresh mint leaves juice with 1 teaspoon lemon juice and one tablespoon honey. Take 3 times a day for relief from piles.
- Boil a mashed ripe banana in one tea cup milk and take 2-3 times a day. Apply a crushed onion, which has been skinned and roasted, to dry and bleeding piles.

Appendix–1

Understanding Diseases

Alzheimer's Disease is an oft-feared illness. When someone over the age of 60 begins to forget where he or she left a set of keys, they may begin to wonder whether it's the first sign of Alzheimer's. Likewise, when an ageing parent can't seem to find the right words in normal conversation, an adult child may also fear the onset of Alzheimer's. There are symptoms of Alzheimer's that differ from symptoms of normal ageing. Distinguishing between the two can be difficult, as they often overlap.

Amenorrhoea is the absence of a menstrual period in a woman of reproductive age. Physiologic states of amenorrhoea are seen during pregnancy and lactation (breastfeeding), the latter also forming the basis of a form of contraception known as the lactational amenorrhoea. There is absence of menses during childhood and after menopause.

Cushing's Syndrome is a hormonal disorder caused by prolonged exposure of the body's tissues to high levels of the hormone cortisol. Cushing's syndrome occurs when the body's tissues are exposed to excessive levels of cortisol for long periods of time. Many people suffer the symptoms of Cushing's syndrome because they take glucocorticoid hormones such as prednisone for asthma, rheumatoid arthritis, lupus and other inflammatory diseases, or for immunosuppression after transplantation. Cortisol performs vital tasks in the body. It helps maintain blood pressure and cardiovascular function, reduces the immune system's inflammatory response, balances the effects of insulin in breaking down sugar for energy, and regulates the metabolism of proteins, carbohydrates, and fats. One of cortisol's most important jobs is to help the body respond to stress.

For this reason, women in their last 3 months of pregnancy and highly trained athletes normally have high levels of the hormone. People suffering from depression, alcoholism, malnutrition and panic disorders also have increased cortisol levels.

Circumcision refers to the surgical removal of the foreskin of the penis.

Dementia (from Latin de- "apart, away," + mens (genitive mentis) "mind") is progressive decline in cognitive function due to damage or disease in the brain beyond what might be expected from normal ageing. Particularly affected areas may be memory, attention, language and problem solving, although particularly in the later stages of the condition, affected persons may be disoriented in time (not knowing what day, week, month or year it is), place (not knowing where they are) and person (not knowing who they are). Symptoms of dementia can be classified as either reversible or irreversible depending upon the etiology of the disease. Less than 10 percent of all dementias are reversible. Dementia is a non-specific term that encompasses many disease processes, just as fever is attributable to many etiologies.

Endoscopy enables the physician to look inside the esophagus, stomach, and duodenum (first part of the small intestine). The procedure might be used to discover the reason for swallowing difficulties, nausea, vomiting, reflux, bleeding, indigestion, abdominal pain, or chest pain.

Galactosemia is a rare genetic metabolic disorder which affects an individual's ability to properly digest the sugar galactose. Lactose in food (such as dairy products) is broken down by the body into glucose and galactose. Normally, galactose is then converted into glucose by the enzyme GALT (galactose-1-phosphate uridylyltransferase). In individuals with galactosemia, GALT activity is severely diminished, leading to toxic levels of galactose to build up in the blood, resulting in hepatomegaly (an enlarged liver), renal failure, cataracts, and brain damage. Without treatment, mortality in infants with galactosemia is about 75 percent.

Parkinson's disease is a movement disorder that is chronic and progressive, meaning that symptoms continue and worsen over time. Approximately 15 percent of people with Parkinson's are diagnosed before the age of 40, incidence increases with age. The cause is unknown, there are many treatment options such as medication and surgery to manage the symptoms.

Parkinson's disease occurs when a group of cells in an area of the brain called the substantia nigra begin to malfunction and die. These cells in the substantia nigra produce a chemical called dopamine. Dopamine is a neurotransmitter, or chemical messenger, that sends information to the parts of the brain that control movement and coordination. When a person has Parkinson's disease, their dopamine-producing cells begin to die and the amount of dopamine produced in the brain decreases. Messages from the brain telling the body how and when to move are therefore delivered more slowly, leaving a person incapable of initiating and controlling movements in a normal way. Parkinson's disease can also cause several different symptoms. The specific group of symptoms that an individual experience varies from person to person. Some of the most common symptoms of Parkinson's disease are:

- Tremor of the hands, arms, legs, jaw and face
- Rigidity or stiffness of the limbs and trunk
- Bradykinesia or slowness of movement
- Postural instability or impaired balance and coordination

Thalassemia is the name of a group of genetic blood disorders. Hemoglobin is the oxygen-carrying component of the red blood cells. It consists of two different proteins, an alpha and a beta. If the body doesn't produce enough of either of these two proteins, the red blood cells do not form properly and cannot carry sufficient oxygen. The result is anemia that begins in early childhood and lasts throughout life.

Since thalassemia is not a single disorder but a group of related disorders that affect the human body in similar ways, it is important to understand the differences between the various types of thalassemia.

Wilson's disease causes the body to retain copper. The liver of a person who has Wilson's disease does not release copper into bile as it should. Bile is a liquid produced by the liver that helps with digestion. As the intestines absorb copper from food, the copper builds up in the liver and injures liver tissue. Eventually, the damage causes the liver to release the copper directly into the bloodstream, which carries the copper throughout the body. The copper buildup leads to damage in the kidneys, brain, and eyes. If not treated, Wilson's disease can cause severe brain damage, liver failure, and death. Wilson's disease is hereditary.

Hodgkin's disease (HD) is the major tumor in a group known as malignant lymphomas. Most often HD starts in B-cell lymphocytes located in lymph nodes in the neck area, although any lymph node may be the site of initial disease.

Appendix–2

The pH Scale

The concentration of hydrogen ions is commonly expressed in terms of the pH scale. Low pH corresponds to high hydrogen ion concentration and vice versa. pH is measured on a scale from 0 to 14.0. An environment with a pH of 7.0 is exactly neutral—neither acid nor alkaline. Foods with a pH below 7.0 are acidic; pH above 7.0 is alkaline. The lower the pH, the higher the acidity; the higher the pH, the lower the acidity.

Concentration of Hydrogen ions compared to distilled water		Examples of solutions at this pH
10,000,000	pH = 0	Battery acid, Strong Hydrofluoric Acid
1,000,000	pH = 1	Hydrochloric acid secreated by stomach lining
100,000	pH = 2	Lemon Juice, Gastric Acid Vineger
10,000	pH = 3	Grapefruit, Orance Juice, Soda
1,000	pH = 4	Acid rain Tomato Juice
100	pH = 5	Soft drinking water Black Coffee
10	pH = 6	Urine Saliva
1	pH = 7	"Pure" water
1/10	pH = 8	Sea water
1/100	pH = 9	Baking soda
1/1,000	pH = 10	Great Salt Lake
1/10,000	pH = 11	Milk of Magnesia Ammonia solution
1/100,000	pH = 12	Soapy water
1/1,000,000	pH = 13	Bleaches Oven cleaner
1/10,000,000	pH = 14	Liquid drain cleaner

Appendix–3

Glossary

Additives (Food Additives)

Additives may be defined as any natural or synthetic material, other than the basic raw ingredients, which are used in the production of a food item to enhance the final product.

Alpha-Carotene

A type of carotenoid found in carrots which provides the health benefit of neutralizing free radicals that may cause damage to cells.

Alzheimer's Disease

It is an oft-feared illness. When someone over the age of 60 begins to forget where he or she left a set of keys, they may begin to wonder whether it's the first sign of Alzheimer's. Likewise, when an ageing parent can't seem to find the right words in normal conversation, an adult child may also fear the onset of Alzheimer's. There are symptoms of Alzheimer's that differ from symptoms of normal ageing. Distinguishing between the two can be difficult, as they often overlap.

Amino Acids

Amino acids are the building blocks of proteins. Chemically, these are organic compounds containing an amino (NH2) group and a carboxyl (COOH) group. Amino acids are classified as essential, nonessential and conditionally essential. If body synthesis is inadequate to meet metabolic need, an amino acid is classified as essential and must be supplied as part of the diet. Essential amino acids include leucine, isoleucine, valine, tryptophan, phenylalanine, methionine, threonine, lysine, histidine and possibly arginine. Nonessential amino acids can be synthesized by the body in adequate amounts, and include alanine, aspartic acid, asparagine, glutamic acid, glutamine, glycine, proline and serine. Conditionally essential amino acids become essential under certain clinical conditions.

Amenorrhoea

Amenorrhoea is the absence of menstrual period in a woman of reproductive age. Physiological states of amenorrhoea are seen during pregnancy and lactation.

Anemia

Anemia is a condition in which a deficiency in the size or number of erythrocytes (red blood cells) or the amount of hemoglobin they contain limits the exchange of oxygen and carbon dioxide between the blood and the tissue cells. Most anemia are caused by a lack of nutrients required for normal erythrocyte synthesis, principally iron, vitamin B_{12}, and folic acid. Others result from a variety of conditions, such as hemorrhage, genetic abnormalities, chronic disease states or drug toxicity.

Anorexia Nervosa

An eating disorder characterized by refusal to eat, to maintain a minimally normal weight for height and age. The condition includes weight loss leading to maintenance of body weight 15 percent below normal; an intense fear of weight gain or becoming fat, despite the individual's underweight status; a disturbance in the self-awareness of one's own body weight or shape; and in females, the absence of at least three consecutive menstrual cycles that would otherwise be expected to occur.

Antibody

Antibodies are the proteins produced by the immune system of humans and higher animals in response to the presence of a specific antigen.

Anticarcinogens

Substances, which inhibit the formation of cancers or the growth of tumors. More than 600 chemicals are claimed to be anti-cancer agents. These range from natural chemical constituent present in garlic, broccoli, cabbage and green tea to manmade antioxidants, such as butylated hydroxyanisole (BHA) and derivatives of retinoic acid.

Antigen

A foreign substance (almost always a protein) that, when introduced into the body, stimulates an immune response.

Antioxidant

Antioxidants protect key cell components by neutralizing the damaging effects of "free radicals," natural byproducts of cell metabolism. Free radicals form when oxygen is metabolized, or burned by the body. They travel through cells, disrupting the structure of other molecules, causing cellular damage. Such cell damage is believed to contribute to ageing and various health problems.

Ascorbic Acid

Also known as vitamin C, it is essential for the development and maintenance of connective tissue. Vitamin C speeds the production of new cells in wound healing and it is an antioxidant that keeps free radicals from hooking up with other molecules to form damaging compounds that might attack tissue. Vitamin C protects the immune system, helps fight off infections, reduces the severity of allergic reactions and plays a role in the synthesis of hormones and other body chemicals. Green peppers, broccoli, citrus fruits, tomatoes, strawberries, and other fresh fruits and vegetables are good sources of vitamin C.

Aspartame

Aspartame is a low-calorie sweetener used in a variety of foods and beverages and as a tabletop sweetener. It is about 200 times sweeter than sugar. Aspartame is made by joining two protein components, aspartic acid and phenylalanine.

Asthma

Asthma is a chronic medical condition. It results when irritants (or trigger substances) cause swelling of the tissues in the air passage of the lungs, making it difficult to breathe. Typical symptoms of asthma include wheezing, shortness of breath and coughing.

Atherosclerosis

A condition that exists when too much cholesterol builds up in the blood and accumulates in the walls of the blood vessels.

Anabolism

It is the process of building up of body substances e.g. proteins from amino acids.

Basal Metabolism

Basal metabolism is the energy a body burns when completely at rest to keep involuntary body processes going. These processes include heartbeat, breathing, generating body heat, perspiring to keep cool, and transmitting messages to the brain. For a sedentary person, BMR accounts for about 60–70 percent of daily energy expenditure, the remaining 30–40 percent is from physical activity and from body heat produced after a meal. Physical activity is responsible for as much as 50–60 percent of the total energy expenditure in people who include frequent aerobic activity into their lifestyles

Balanced Diet

A balanced diet is one that contains different type of foods in such quantities and proportions that the need for calories, minerals, vitamins and other nutrients is adequately met. A balanced diet should provide around 60–70 percent of total calories from carbohydrates, 10–12 percent from protein and 20–25 percent from fat.

Beta-Carotene

A type of carotenoid found in various fruits and vegetables.

Bulimia Nervosa

An eating disorder characterized by rapid consumption of a large amount of food in a short period of time, with a sense of lack of control during the episode and self-evaluation unduly influenced by body weight and shape. There are two forms of the condition, purging and non-purging. The first type regularly engages in purging through self-induced vomiting or the excessive use of laxatives or diuretics. Alternatively, the non-purging type controls weight through strict dieting, fasting or excessive exercise.

Carcinogen

It is a substance that can cause cancer.

Calorie

A calorie is the amount of heat required to raise the temperature of one kilogram of water through one degree at 15 Celsius (c).

Catabolism

It is the process of breaking down of body substances e.g. during fever, burn, injury etc.

Cyclamate

A sweetener, which is 30 times sweeter than sucrose, calorie free and heat stable and works synergistically with other sweeteners. It is approved for tabletop use in Canada and more than 50 countries in Europe, Asia, South America and Africa. Since 1970, however, the use of cyclamate has been banned in the United States on the basis of a study that suggested that cyclamates may be related to the development of bladder tumors in rats.

Cholesterol

Cholesterol is a soft, waxy substance present in all parts of the body including the nervous system, skin, muscle, liver, intestines and heart. It is both made by the body and obtained from animal products in the diet. Cholesterol is manufactured in the liver for normal body functions including the production of hormones, bile acid and Vitamin D.

Dietetics

It is the science that deals with the adequacy of diets during normal life cycle and modifications during diseases.

Diet-induced Thermogenesis (Specific Dynamic Action (SDA))

Diet-induced thermogenesis is the energy used by the body to digest, absorb, transport and metabolize the food that a person eats. This is usually equal to about 10 percent of the calories that we eat.

Enzyme

Enzymes are complex proteins that assist or enable chemical reactions to occur. "Digestive" enzymes, for example, help the body break food down into chemical compounds that can more easily be absorbed. Thousands of different enzymes are produced by the body.

Enriched Grains

These are refined grain products to which key nutrients usually minerals (Iron) and vitamins e.g. A, C, D, Thiamine, B2 and B3 have been added.

Food Allergen

A food allergen is the part of a food (a protein) that stimulates the immune system of food allergic individuals. A single food can contain multiple food allergens.

Food Allergy

A food allergy is any adverse reaction to a harmless food or food component (a protein) that involves the body's immune system.

Food

Food can be defined as anything solid and liquid which when swallowed, digested and assimilated in the body keeps it well.

Flavonoids (bioflavinoids): Flavonoids are water-soluble pigments that are found in many plants. Many of the flavonoids serve as antioxidants or play other important roles in maintaining the health of body.

Glycogenesis

It is the formation of glycogen from glucose.

Glycogenolysis

Glycogen is converted back to glucose.

Gluconeogenesis

It is the process of synthesizing glucose from non-carbohydrate sources.

Glycemic Index (GI)

The Glycemic Index is a dietary index that's used to rank carbohydrate-based foods. The Glycemic Index predicts the rate at which the ingested food will increase blood sugar levels.

Health

Health is defined as the "state of complete physical, mental and social well being and not merely the absence of disease and infirmity".

Ligament

It is a dense fibrous connective tissue, which helps to join one bone to another bone, the joints and also hold them in position.

Menu Planning

It is a process of planning and scheduling intake of meals for a general or specific individual requirements.

Nutrition

Nutrition is the branch of science, which deals with the study of nutrients, their action, interaction and balance in relationship to health and disease.

Nutrients

Nutrients are the constituents in food that must be supplied to the body in suitable amounts or nutrients are the chemical components of food that supply nourishment to the body.

Nutritional Status

It is the condition/state of health of an individual as influenced by the utilization of nutrients in the body.

Nutrient Requirement

Nutrient requirement can be defined as the minimum amount of the absorbed nutrient that is necessary for maintaining the normal physiological functions of the body.

Optimum Nutrition

Optimum nutrition means that a person is receiving and utilizing essential nutrients in proportions as required by the body while also providing a reserve.

Prebiotics

Prebiotics are defined as non-digestible food ingredients that may beneficially affect the host by selectively stimulating the growth and/or the activity of a limited number of bacteria in the colon.

Probiotics

Cultures of beneficial microorganisms fed to live stock to improve digestion and improve health or microorganism that have beneficial effects on their host.These are the dietary supplements containing potentially beneficial bacteria and yeasts.

Proteinuria

Urine output is less than 1 ml/kg/h in infants, less than 0.5ml/kg/h in children and less than 400 ml/d in adults.

Syndrome X

Syndrome X refers to a group of health problems that include, insulin resistance, abnormal fat in the blood, over weight and high blood pressure.

Sugar Alcohol

Sugar alcohols, sometimes called polyols, are a class of carbohydrates that are more slowly or incompletely absorbed by the human digestive system than sugars. Common sugar alcohols include sorbitol, mannitol, maltitol, and xylitol. Sugar alcohols contribute less calories to the diet than most other types of carbohydrates, but may cause digestive discomfort.

Toxemia

A condition in which toxins move into the blood stream.

Tendon

It is a very thick dense and strong connective tissue mainly composed of white tissue, helps to join a muscle to a bone.

Uremia

Urea is retained in the blood, because of kidney diseases.

Whole grain

The term whole grain is used for food products such as flours, bread or cereals that are produced from unrefined grains, which is grain that still retains its outer bran layers and inner germ endosperm and their nutrients i.e. dietary fibre, mineral, vitamins.

Appendix-4

Various Food Exchange List

Milk Exchange List

(On an average, one milk exchange provides 8 g protein, 12 g carbohydrate, 10 g fat, 170 kcal)

Food	Amount (g)	Protein (g)	Carbo-hydrate (g)	Fat (g)	Energy (kcal)
Cow's milk	250	8	11.5	103	168
Buffalo's milk	185	8	9.3	16.3	216
Skim milk	320	8	14.7	Neg.	93
Skim milk powder	21	8	10.7	Neg.	75
Whole milk powder	31	8	11.8	8.0	154
Butter milk	1000	8	5.0	11.0	155
Curd	258	8	7.7	10.3	155
Cheese	33	8	2.1	8.2	115
Khoa,buffalo	55	8	11.3	17.2	231
Khoa,cow	40	8	8	10.4	165
Khoa, skim milk	36	8	8.7	0.5	70

Meat Exchange List

(On an average one meat exchange provides 7 g protein, 5 g fat, negligible carbohydrate, 70 kcal)

Food	Amount (g)	Protein (g)	Carbo-hydrate (g)	Fat (g)	Energy (kcal)
Egg	53	7	-	7	81
Fowl	27	7	-	0.2	29
Goat meat	32	7	-	1.2	38
Mutton muscle	38	7	-	5.1	73
Pork	37	7	-	1.7	43
Hilsa	32	7	-	6.2	87
Katla	35	7	-	0.8	39
Prawn	37	7	-	0.4	32
Rohu	42	7	-	0.6	41
Cheese	29	7	1.8	7.3	101
Channa, cow	38	7	0.46	7.9	101
Channa, buffalo	52	7	4.11	1.2	152

Pulse Exchange List

(On an average one pulse exchange provides 7 g protein, negligible fat, 17 g carbohydrate, 100 kcal)

Food	Amount (g)	Protein (g)	Carbo-hydrate (g)	Fat (g)	Energy (kcal)
Bengal gram (roasted)	31	7	1.6	18	114
Bengal gram (whole)	41	7	2.2	25	148
Bengal gram dal	34	7	1.8	20	125
Black gram dal	29	7	0.4	17	101
Cowpea (lobia)	29	7	0.3	16	94
Green gram, whole	29	7	0.4	16	97
Green gram, dal	28	7	0.3	17	101
Lentil	29	7	0.2	16	96
Peas, dry	35	7	04	20	110
Rajmah	30	7	05	18	105
Red gram dal	31	7	0.5	18	104
Soybean	16	7	32	34	70
Moth bean	30	7	0.3	17	99

Cereal/Starch Exchange list

(On an average one cereal exchange provides 15 g carbohydrate, 2 g protein, negligible fat and 70 kcal)

Food	Amount (g)	Protein (g)	Carbo-hydrate (g)	Fat (g)	Energy (kcal)
Bajra	22	15	2.6	-	79
Barley	22	15	2.5	-	74
Bread, white	29	15	2.3	-	71
Bread, brown	31	15	2.7	-	76
Biscuit, salty	28	15	1.8	-	156
Biscuit, sweet	21	15	1.3	-	156
Jowar	21	15	2.2	-	73
Maize, dry	23	15	2.6	-	79
Maize,tender	61	15	2.9	-	76
Oat meal	24	15	3.3	-	90
Ragi	21	15	1.5	-	69
Rice, raw milled	19	15	1.3	-	66
Rice flakes	19	15	1.3	-	66
Rice, puffed	20	15	1.5	-	65
Semolina	20	15	2.1	-	70
Bulgar wheat	19	15	1.6	-	68
Wheat flour, whole	22	15	2.7	-	75
Wheat flour, refined	20	15	2.2	-	70
Vermicelli	19	15	1.7	-	67
Lotus stem	75	15	1.2	-	70
Colocasia, fresh	71	15	2.1	-	69
Potato	66	15	1.0	-	64
Potato, sweet	53	15	0.6	-	64
Yam	58	15	0.8	-	64

Vegetable A exchange list

(1 exchange of vegetable A is 100 g and provides up to 3 g carbohydrate, negligible protein and fat)

Food	% Carbohydrate
Bathua leaves	2.9
Bottle gourd	2.5
Cucumber	2.5
Ghosla (ghia tori)	2.9
Lettuce	2.5
Mustard leaves	3.2
Parwal	2.2
Raddish leaves	2.4
Raddish, white	3.4
Ridge gourd	3.4
Snake gourd	3.3
Spinach	2.9
Tinda	3.4

Vegetable B exchange

(On an average vegetable B exchange provides 7 g carbohydrate, 2g protein, negligible fat and 40 kcals)

Food	Weight (g)	Carbohydrate (g)	Protein (g)	Energy (kcal)
Amaranth	115	7	4.6	52
Beetroot	80	7	1.4	34
Bittergourd	167	7	2.7	42
Brinjal	175	7	2.7	42
Broad beans	97	7	4.4	47
Cabbage	152	7	2.7	41
Capsicum	162	7	2.1	39
Carrot	66	7	0.6	32
Cauliflower	175	7	4.5	53
Colocasia leaves	103	7	4.3	58
Coriander leaves	111	7	3.7	40
Drumstick	192	7	4.8	48
Fenugreek leaves	117	7	3.1	57
French beans	156	7	2.6	41
Jack fruit	75	7	1.9	38
Knol khol	184	7	22.1	38
Lady's finger	109	7	2.0	38
Mint leaves	121	7	5.0	58
Onion, small	56	7	1.0	33
Plantain, green	50	7	0.7	32
Peas	44	7	3.2	41
Pumpkin	152	7	2.1	38
Tomato, ripe	194	7	1.7	30
Turnip	113	7	0.6	33
Mushroom	163	7	2.3	47

Fruit exchange list

(On an average one fruit exchange provides, 10 g carbohydrate, negligible protein and fat, 40 kcals)

Food	Amount (g)	Carbohydrate (g)	Energy (kcal)
Amla	74	10	42
Apricot, fresh	86	10	46
Apple	75	10	44
Banana	37	10	42
Cherries	72	10	46
Dates, fresh	30	10	43
Dates, dry	13	10	41
Grape Fruit	143	10	46
Grapes	61	10	41
Guava	80	10	45
Lemon (Sweet)	92	10	51
Lichi	73	10	44
Lime, sweet (Malta)	128	10	46
Lime,sweet (Musambi)	107	10	46
Loquat	104	10	44
Mango	59	10	44
Orange	92	10	44
Papaya	139	10	44
Pear	84	10	44
Peaches	95	10	48
Pineapple	93	10	43
Plums	90	10	47
Pomegranate	69	10	44
Rasberry	80	10	48
Raisins	13	10	41
Sapota	47	10	46
Water melon	303	10	49
Musk melon	286	10	49

Fat and nuts exchange list

(On an average one fat exchange provides 5 g fat, 45 kcals)

Food	Weight (g)	Fat (g)	Protein- (g)	Carbo-hydrate (g)	Energy (kcal)
Butter	6	5	-	-	45
Ghee	5	5	-	-	45
Hydrogenated oil	5	5	-	-	45
Cooking oil	5	5	-	-	45
Cream	25	5	-	-	50
Almonds	8	5	1.7	0.8	53
Cashewnuts	11	5	2.3	2.5	66
Coconut, dry	8	5	0.3	1.5	53
Coconut, fresh	12	5	0.5	1.6	53
Gingelly seeds	12	5	2.2	3.0	58
Groundnuts, roasted	13	5	3.4	3.5	74
Walnuts	8	5	1.3	0.9	55

Source: Khanna, K. 2003. Textbook of Nutrition and Dietetics, University of Delhi.

Appendix-5

Food composition tables

Cereal and Cereal Products														
Name of the food	Moisture (gm)	Protein (gm)	Fat (gm)	Minerals (gm)	Fibre (gm)	Carbohydrates (gm)	Energy (kcal)	Calcium (mg)	Phosphorus (mg)	Iron (mg)	Carotene (mg)	Thiamine (mg)	Riboflavin (mg)	Niacin (mg)
Bajra	12.4	11.6	5	2.3	1.2	67.5	361	42	296	5	132	0.33	0.25	2.3
Jowar	11.9	10.4	1.9	1.6	1.6	72.6	349	25	222	5.8	47	0.37	0.13	3.1
Maize, dry	14.9	11.1	3.6	1.5	2.7	66.2	342	10	348	2	90	0.42	0.1	1.8
Maize, tender	67.1	4.7	0.9	0.8	1.9	24.6	125	9	121	1.1	32	0.11	0.17	0.6
Ragi	13.1	7.3	1.3	2.7	3.6	72	328	344	283	6.4	42	0.42	0.19	1.1
Rice parboiled handpounded	12.6	8.5	0.6	0.9	-	77.4	349	10	280	2.8	9	0.27	0.12	4
Rice parboiled milled	13.3	6.4	0.4	0.7	0.2	79	346	9	143	4	-	0.21	0.05	3.8
Rice raw hand-pounded	13.3	7.5	1	0.9	0.6	76.7	346	10	190	3.2	2	0.21	0.16	3.9
Rice raw milled	13.7	6.8	0.5	0.6	0.2	78.2	345	10	160	3.1	0	0.06	.060	1.9

Continued

Cereal and Cereal Products

Name of the food	Moisture (gm)	Protein (gm)	Fat (gm)	Minerals (gm)	Fibre (gm)	Carbohydrates (gm)	Energy (kcal)	Calcium (mg)	Phosphorus (mg)	Iron (mg)	Carotene (mg)	Thiamine (mg)	Riboflavin (mg)	Niacin (mg)
Rice bran	11	13.5	16.2	6.6	4.3	48.4	393	67	1410	35	-	2.1	0.48	-
Rice flakes	12.2	6.6	1.2	2	0.7	77.3	346	20	238	20	0	0.21	0.05	4
Rice puffed	14.7	7.5	0.1	3.8	0.3	73.6	325	23	150	6.6	0	0.21	0.01	4.1
Sewai	11.7	7.7	4.7	1.5	7.6	67	341	17	220	5.2	0	0.3	0.09	3.2
Sanwa millet	11.9	6.2	2.2	4.4	9.8	65.5	307	20	280	2.9	0			4.2
Semolina	-	10.4	0.8	-	0.2	74.8	348	16	102	1.6	-	0.12	0.03	1.06
Wheat whole	12.8	11.8	1.5	1.5	1.2	71.2	346	41	306	4.9	64	0.45	0.17	5.5
Wheatflour whole	12.2	12.1	1.7	2.7	1.9	69.4	341	48	355	11.5	29	0.49	0.17	4.3
Wheatflour refined	13.3	11	0.9	0.6	0.3	73.9	348	23	121	2.5	25	0.12	0.07	2.4
Wheat-germ	5.2	29.2	7.4	3.5	1.4	53.3	397	40	846	6	-	1.4	0.54	2.9
Vermicelli	11.7	8.7	0.4	0.7	0.2	78.3	352	22	92	2	0	0.19	0.05	1.8

Pulses and Legumes													
Name of the food	Moisture (gm)	Protein (gm)	Fat (gm)	Minerals (gm)	Fibre (gm)	Carbohydrates (gm)	Energy (kcal)	Calcium (mg)	Phosphorus (mg)	Iron (mg)	Carotene (mg)	Thiamine (mg)	Riboflavin (mg)	Niacin (mg)
Bengal gram whole	9.8	17.1	5.3	3	3.9	60.9	360	202	312	10.2	189	0.3	0.15	2.9
Bengal gram dal	9.9	20.8	5.6	2.7	1.2	59.8	372	56	331	9.1	129	0.48	0.18	2.4
Bengal gram roasted	10.7	22.5	5.2	2.5	1	58.1	369	58	340	9.5	113	0.2	-	1.3
Black gram dal	10.9	24	1.4	3.2	0.9	59.6	347	154	385	9.1	38	0.42	0.2	2
Cowpea	13.4	24.1	1	3.2	3.8	54.5	323	77	414	5.9	12	0.51	0.2	1.3
Fieldbean dry	9.6	24.9	0.8	3.2	1.4	60.1	347	60	433	2.7	0	0.52	0.16	1.8
Green gram whole	10.4	24	1.3	3.5	4.1	56.7	334	124	326	7.3	94	0.47	0.27	2.1
Green gram dal	10.1	24.5	1.2	3.5	0.8	59.9	348	75	405	8.5	49	0.47	0.21	2.4
Lentil	12.4	25.1	0.7	2.1	0.7	59	343	69	293	4.8	270	0.45	0.2	2.6

Continued

Pulses and Legumes														
Name of the food	Moisture (gm)	Protein (gm)	Fat (gm)	Minerals (gm)	Fibre (gm)	Carbohydrates (gm)	Energy (kcal)	Calcium (mg)	Phosphorus (mg)	Iron (mg)	Carotene (mg)	Thiamine (mg)	Riboflavin (mg)	Niacin (mg)
Moth-beans	10.8	23.6	1.1	3.5	4.5	56.5	330	202	230	9.5	9	0.45	0.09	1.5
Peas dry	16	19.7	1.1	2.2	4.5	56.5	315	75	298	5.1	39	0.47	0.19	3.4
Peas roasted	10.1	22.9	1.4	2.4	4.4	58.5	340	81	345	6.4	18	0.47	0.21	3.5
Rajma	12	22.9	1.3	3.2		60.6	346	260	410	5.8	-	-	-	-
Redgram dal	13.4	22.3	1.7	3.5	1.5	57.6	335	73	304	5.8	132	0.45	0.19	2.9
Soybeans	8.1	43.2	19.5	4.6	3.7	20.9	432	240	690	11.5	426	0.73	0.39	3.2

Leafy Vegetables														
Name of the food	Moisture (gm)	Protein (gm)	Fat (gm)	Minerals (gm)	Fibre (gm)	Carbohydrates (gm)	Energy (kcal)	Calcium (mg)	Phosphorus (mg)	Iron (mg)	Carotene (mg)	Thiamine (mg)	Riboflavin (mg)	Niacin (mg)
Amaranth tender	85.7	4	0.5	2.7	1	6.1	45	397	83	25.5	5520	0.03	0.3	1.2
Ambat chukka	95.2	1.6	0.3	0.9	0.6	1.4	15	63	17	8.7	3660	0.03	0.06	0.2
Cabbage	91.9	1.8	1	0.6	1	4.6	27	39	44	0.8	120	0.06	0.09	0.4
Cauliflower green	80.0	5.9	1.3	3.2	2	7.6	66	626	107	40	-	-	-	-
Celery leaves	88.0	6.3	0.6	2.1	1.4	1.6	37	230	140	6.3	3990	0	0.11	1.2
Colocasia back	78.8	6.8	0.2	2.5	1.8	8.1	77	460	125	38.7	12000	0.06	0.45	1.9
Colocasia leaves green	82.7	3.9	1.5	2.2	29	6.8	56	227	82	10	10278	0.22	0.26	1.1
Colocasia leaves dry	9.3	13.7	5.9	13	16	42.3	277	1546	308	-	-	-	-	-
Coriander leaves	86.3	3.3	0.6	2.3	1.2	6.3	44	184	71	18.5	6918	0.05	0.06	0.8
Cowpea leaves	89	3.4	0.7	1.6	1.2	4.1	38	290	58	20.1	6072	0.05	0.18	0.6

Continued

Leafy Vegetables														
Name of the food	Moisture (gm)	Protein (gm)	Fat (gm)	Minerals (gm)	Fibre (gm)	Carbohydrates (gm)	Energy (kcal)	Calcium (mg)	Phosphorus (mg)	Iron (mg)	Carotene (mg)	Thiamine (mg)	Riboflavin (mg)	Niacin (mg)
Curry leaves	63.8	6.1	0.1	4	6.4	18.7	108	830	57	7	7560	0.08	0.21	2.3
Drumstick leaves	75.9	6.7	1.7	2.3	0.9	12.5	92	440	70	7	6780	0.06	0.05	0.8
Fenugreek leaves	86.1	4.4	0.9	1.5	1.1	6	49	395	51	16.5	2340	0.04	0.31	0.8
Knoll-khol green	86.7	3.5	0.4	1.2	1.8	6.4	43	740	50	13.3	4146	0.25	-	3
Lettuce	93.4	2.1	0.3	1.2	0.5	2.5	21	50	28	2.4	990	0.09	0.13	0.5
Mayalu	90.8	2.8	0.4	1.8	-	4.2	32	200	35	10	7440	0.03	0.16	0.5
Mint leaves	84.9	2.8	0.6	1.9	2	5.8	48	200	62	15.6	1620	0.05	0.26	1
Mustard leaves	89.8	4	0.6	1.6	0.8	3.2	34	155	26	16.3	2622	0.03	-	-
Radish leaves	90.8	3.8	0.4	1.6	1	2.4	28	265	59	3.6	5295	0.18	0.47	-
Shepu	88	3	0.5	2.2	1.1	5.2	37	190	42	17.4	7182	0.03	0.13	0.2
Spinach	92.1	2	0.7	1.7	0.6	2.9	26	73	21	10.9	5580	0.03	0.26	0.5
Tamarind leaves tender	70.5	5.8	2.1	1.5	1.9	18.2	115	101	140	5.2	250	0.24	0.17	4.1

Roots and Tubers														
Name of the food	Moisture (gm)	Protein (gm)	Fat (gm)	Minerals (gm)	Fibre (gm)	Carbohydrates (gm)	Energy (kcal)	Calcium (mg)	Phosphorus (mg)	Iron (mg)	Carotene (mg)	Thiamine (mg)	Riboflavin (mg)	Niacin (mg)
Arwa gadda	74.3	1.4	0.1	0.6		23.6	101	30	20	2.2	-	-	-	-
Banana rhizome	85.1	0.4	0.2	1.4	1.1	11.8	51	25	10	1.1	16	0	0.03	0.2
Beet root	87.7	1.7	0.1	0.8	0.9	8.8	43	18.3	55	1	0	0.04	0.09	0.4
Carrot	86	0.9	0.2	1.1	1.2	10.6	48	80	530	2.2	1890	0.04	0.02	0.6
Colocasia	73.1	3	0.1	1.7	1	21.1	97	40	140	1.7	24	0.09	0.03	0.4
Onion big	86.6	1.2	0.1	0.4	0.6	11.1	50	46.9	50	0.7	0	0.08	0.01	0.4
Onion small	84.3	1.8	0.1	0.6	0.6	12.6	59	40	60	1.2	15	0.08	0.02	0.5
Potato	74.7	1.6	0.1	0.6	0.4	22.6	97	10	40	0.7	24	0.1	0.01	1.2
Radish pink	90.8	0.6	0.3	0.9	0.6	6.8	32	50	20	0.5	3	0.06	0.02	0.4
Radish white	94.4	0.7	0.1	0.6	0.8	3.4	17	35	22	0.4	3	0.06	0.02	0.5
Sweet potato	68.5	1.2	0.3	1	0.8	28.2	120	46	50	0.8	6	0.08	0.04	0.7
Tapioca	59.4	0.7	0.2	1	0.6	38.1	157	50	40	0.9	-	0.05	0.1	0.3
Yam elephant	78.7	1.2	0.1	0.8	0.8	18.4	79	50	34	0.6	260	0.06	0.07	0.7
Yam ordinary	69.9	0.4	0.1	1.6	1	26	111	35	20	1.3	78	0.07	-	0.7

Other Vegetables														
Name of the food	Moisture (gm)	Protein (gm)	Fat (gm)	Minerals (gm)	Fibre (gm)	Carbohydrates (gm)	Energy (kcal)	Calcium (mg)	Phosphorus (mg)	Iron (mg)	Carotene (mg)	Thiamine (mg)	Riboflavin (mg)	Niacin (mg)
Ash gourd	96.5	0.4	0.1	0.3	0.8	1.9	10	30	20	0.8	0	0.06	0.01	0.04
Beans scarlet	58.3	7.4	1	1.6	1.9	29.8	158	50	160	2.6	34	0.34	0.19	0
Bitter gourd	92.4	1.6	0.2	0.8	0.8	4.2	25	20	70	1.8	126	0.07	0.09	0.5
Bitter gourd small	83.2	2.1	1	1.4	1.7	10.6	60	23	38	2	126	0.07	0.06	0.4
Bottle gourd	96.1	0.2	0.1	0.5	2.5	2.5	12	20	10	0.7	0	0.03	0.01	0.2
Brinjal	92.7	1.4	0.3	0.3	1.3	4	24	18	47	0.9	74	0.04	0.11	0.9
Broad beans	85.4	4.5	0.1	0.8	2	7.2	48	50	64	1.4	9	0.08	-	0.8
Cauliflower	90.8	2.6	0.4	1	1.2	4	30	33	57	1.5	30	0.04	0.1	1
Cluster beans	81	3.2	0.4	1.4	3.2	10.8	16	130	57	4.5	198	0.09	0.03	0.6
Colocasia stem	94	0.3	0.3	1.2	0.6	3.6	18	60	20	0.5	104	0.07	0.07	0.1

Continued

Other Vegetables

Name of the food	Moisture (gm)	Protein (gm)	Fat (gm)	Minerals (gm)	Fibre (gm) (gm)	Carbohydrates (gm)	Energy (kcal)	Calcium (mg)	Phosphorus (mg)	Iron (mg) (mg)	Carotene (mg)	Thiamine (mg)	Riboflavin (mg)	Niacin (mg)
Knoll-khol	92.7	1.1	0.2	0.7	1.5	3.8	21	20	35	0.4	21	0.05	0.09	0.5
Ladies finger	89.6	1.9	0.2	0.7	1.2	6.4	25	66	56	1.5	52	0.07	0.1	0.6
Mango green	87.5	0.7	0.1	0.4	1.2	10.1	44	10	19	5.4	90	0.05	0.01	0.2
Papaya green	92	0.7	0.2	0.5	0.9	5.7	27	28	40	0.9	0	0.01	0.01	0.1
Parvar	92	2	0.3	0.5	3	2.2	20	30	40	1.7	153	0.05	0.06	0.5
Peas	72.1	7.2	0.1	0.8	4	15.9	93	20	139	1.5	83	0.25	0.01	0.8
Pink beans	86.8	3.1	0.4	0.6	2.1	7	44	54	70	1.5	453	0.06	0.02	0.6
Plantain flower	89.9	1.7	0.7	1.3	1.3	5.1	34	32	42	1.6	27	0.05	0.02	0.4
Plantain green	83.2	1.4	0.2	0.5	0.7	14	64	10	29	0.6	30	0.05	0.02	0.3
Plantain Stem	88.3	0.5	0.1	0.6	0.8	9.7	42	10	10	1.1	0	0.02	0.01	0.2
Pumpkin	92.6	1.4	0.1	0.6	0.7	4.6	25	10	30	0.7	50	0.06	0.04	0.5
Leeks	78.9	1.8	0.1	0.7	1.3	17.2	77	50	70	2.3	18	0.23	-	-

Continued

Other Vegetables														
Name of the food	Moisture (gm)	Protein (gm)	Fat (gm)	Minerals (gm)	Fibre (gm)	Carbohydrates (gm)	Energy (kcal)	Calcium (mg)	Phosphorus (gm)	Iron (mg)	Carotene (mg)	Thiamine (mg)	Riboflavin (mg)	Niacin (mg)
Redgram tender	65.5	9.8	1	1	6.2	16.9	116	57	164	1.1	469	0.32	0.33	3
Ridge gourd	95.2	0.5	0.1	0.3	0.5	3.4	70	18	26	0.5	33	-	0.01	0.2
Snake gourd	94.6	0.5	0.3	0.5	0.8	3.3	18	26	20	0.3	96	0.04	0.06	0.3
Sword beans	87.2	2.7	0.2	0.6	1.5	7.8	44	60	40	2	24	00.8	0.08	0.5
Tinda tender	93.5	1.4	0.2	0.5	1	3.4	21	25	24	0.9	13	.4	0.08	0.3
Tomato green	93.1	1.9	0.1	0.6	0.7	3.6	23	20	36	1.8	192	0.07	0.01	0.4
Vegetable marrow	94.8	0.5	0.1	0.3	0.8	3.5	17	10	30	0.6	-	0.02	0	0.4
Water chestnut fresh	70	4.7	0.3	1.1	0.6	23.3	115	20	150	0.8	12	0.05	0.07	0.6
Water chestnut dry	13.8	13.4	0.8	3.1	-	68.9	336	70	440	24	-	-	-	-

Nuts and Oilseeds														
Name of the food	Moi-sture (gm)	Pro-tein (gm)	Fat (gm)	Mine-rals (gm)	Fibre (gm)	Carbohy-drates (gm)	Energy (kcal)	Calcium (mg)	Phos-phorus (mg)	Iron (mg)	Caro-tene (mg)	Thia-mine (mg)	Ribo-flavin (mg)	Niacin (mg)
Almond	5.2	20.8	58.9	2.9	1.7	10.5	655	230	490	4.5	0	0.24	0.57	4.4
Cashew nut	5.9	21.2	46.9	2.4	1.3	22.3	596	50	450	5	60	0.63	0.19	1.2
Chilgoza	4	13.9	49.3	2.8	1	29	615	91	494	3.6	-	0.32	0.3	3.6
Coconut dry	4.3	6.8	62.3	1.6	6.6	18.4	662	400	210	2.7	0	0.08	0.01	3
Coconut fresh	36.3	4.5	41.6	1	3.6	13	444	10	240	1.7	0	0.05	0.1	0.8
Garden cress seeds	3.2	25.3	24.5	6.4	7.6	33	454	377	723	100	27	0.59	0.61	14
Gingelly seeds	5.3	18.3	43.3	5.2	2.9	25	563	1450	570	10.5	60	1.01	0.34	4.44
Ground nut	3	25.3	40.1	2.4	3.1	26.1	567	90	350	2.8	37	0.9	0.13	20
Ground nut roasted	1.7	26.2	39.8	2.5	3.1	26.7	570	77	370	3.1	0	0.39	0.13	22
Mustard seeds	8.5	20	39.7	4.2	1.8	23.8	541	490	700	7.9	162	0.65	0.26	4
Niger seeds	42	23.9	39	4.9	11	7.1	515	300	224	56.6	-	0.07	0.97	8.4
Oyster nuts	4.4	29.7	63.3	2.6	-	0	689	10	570	4.1	-	-	-	-
Pistachio nuts	5.6	19.8	53.5	2.8	2.1	16.2	626	140	430	7.7	144	0.67	0.28	0.2
Walnuts	45	15.6	64.5	1.8	2.	1	687	100	380	4.8	6	0.45	0.4	1

Fruits

Name of the food	Moisture (gm)	Protein (gm)	Fat (gm)	Minerals (gm)	Fibre (gm)	Carbohydrates (gm)	Energy (kcal)	Calcium (mg)	Phosphorus (mg)	Iron (mg)	Carotene (mg)	Thiamine (mg)	Riboflavin (mg)	Niacin (mg)
Ambada	90.4	0.7	3	0.5	1	4.5	48	36	11	3.9	270	0.02	0.02	0.3
Amla	81.8	0.5	0.1	0.5	3.4	13.7	58	50	20	1.2	9	0.03	0.01	0.2
Apple	84.6	0.2	0.5	0.3	1	13.4	59	10	14	1	0	-	-	0
Apricot fresh	85.3	1	0.3	0.7	1.1	11.6	53	20	25	2.2	2160	0.04	0.13	0.6
Apricot dried	19.4	1.6	0.7	2.8	2.1	73.4	306	110	70	4.6	58	0.22	-	2.3
Banana ripe	70.1	1.2	0.3	0.8	0.4	27.2	116	17	36	0.9	78	0.05	0.08	0.5
Bullocks heart	76.8	1.4	0.2	0.7	5.2	15.7	70	10	10	0.6	67	-	0.07	0.6
Cashew fruit	86.3	0.2	0.1	0.2	0.9	12.3	51	10	10	0.2	23	0.02	0.05	0.4
Cherries red	83.4	1.1	0.5	0.8	0.4	13.8	64	24	25	1.3	0	0.08	0.08	0.03
Currants black	18.4	2.7	0.5	2.2	1	75.2	32	130	110	8.5	21	0.03	0.14	0.4
Dates dried	15.3	2.5	0.4	2.1	3.9	75.8	317	120	50	7.3	26	0.01	0.02	0.9
Dates fresh	59.2	1.2	0.4	1.7	3.7	33.8	144	22	38	-	-	-	-	-
Figs	88.1	1.3	0.2	0.6	2.2	7.6	37	80	30	1	162	0.06	0.05	0.06
Grapes blue	82.2	0.6	0.4	0.9	2.8	13.1	58	20	23	0.5	3	0.04	0.03	0.2

Continued

Fruits														
Name of the food	Moisture (gm)	Protein (gm)	Fat (gm)	Minerals (gm)	Fibre (gm)	Carbohydrates (gm)	Energy (kcal)	Calcium (mg)	Phosphorus (mg)	Iron (mg)	Carotene (mg)	Thiamine (mg)	Riboflavin (mg)	Niacin (mg)
Water melon	95.8	0.2	0.2	0.3	0.2	3.3	16	11	12	7.9	0	0.02	0.04	0.1
Orange	87.6	0.7	0.2	0.3	0.3	10.9	48	26	20	0.32	1104	-	-	-
Orange juice	97.7	0.2	0.1	0.1	-	1.9	9	5	9	0.7	15	0.06	0.02	0.4
Papaya ripe	90.8	0.6	0.1	0.5	0.8	7.2	32	17	13	0.5	66	0.04	0.25	0.2
Peaches	86	1.2	0.3	0.8	1.2	10.5	50	15	41	2.4	0	0.02	0.03	0.5
Pears	86	0.6	0.2	0.3	1	11.9	52	8	15	0.5	28	0.06	0.03	0.2
Pineapple	87.8	0.4	0.1	0.4	0.5	10.8	46	20	9	1.2	18	0.2	0.12	0.1
Pomegranate	78	1.6	0.1	0.7	5.1	14.5	65	10	70	0.3	0	0.06	0.1	0.3
Prunes	85.3	0.5	0.3	0.6	0.5	12.8	56	10	18	-	-	-	-	-
Plum	86.9	0.7	0.5	0.4	0.4	11.1	52	10	12	0.6	166	0.04	0.1	0.3
Raisins	20.2	1.8	0.3	2	1.1	4	308	87	80	7.7	2.4	0.07	0.19	0.7
Raspberry	84.8	1	0.6	0.9	1	11.7	56	40	110	2.3	1248	-	-	0.8
Sapota	73.7	0.7	1.1	0.5	2.6	21.4	98	28	27	2	97	0.02	0.03	0.2
Sitafal	70.5	1.6	0.4	0.9	3.1	23.5	104	17	47	1.5	0	0.07	0.17	1.3
Strawberry	87.8	0.7	0.2	0.4	1.1	9.8	44	30	30	1.8	18	0.03	0.02	0.2
Tomato ripe	94	0.9	0.2	0.5	0.8	3.6	20	48	20	0.4	351	0.12	0.06	0.4
Tree tomato	86.2	1.5	0.2	1.2	4.2	6.7	35	12	46	1	324	0.11	0.06	2.1
Ber	81.6	0.8	0.3	0.3	-	17	74	4	9	1.8	21	0.02	0.05	0.7

Milk and Milk Products

Name of the food	Moi-sture (gm)	Pro-tein (gm)	Fat (gm)	Mine-rals (gm)	Fibre (gm)	Carbohy-drates (gm)	Energy (kcal)	Calcium (mg)	Phos-phorus (mg)	Iron (mg)	Caro-tene (mg)	Thia-mine (mg)	Ribo-flavin (mg)	Niacin (mg)
Buffalo milk	81	4.3	8.8	0.8	-	5	117	210	130	0.2	160	0.04	0.1	0.1
Cow milk	87.5	3.2	4.1	0.8	-	4.4	67	120	90	0.2	174	0.05	0.19	0.1
Goat milk	86.8	3.3	4.5	0.8	-	4.6	72	127	120	0.3	182	0.05	0.04	0.3
Human milk	88	1.1	3.4	0.1	-	7.4	65	28	11	-	137	0.02	0.02	-
Curd cowmilk	89.1	3.1	4	0.8	-	3	60	149	93	0.2	102	0.05	0.16	0.1
Skimmed milk	92.1	2.5	0.1	0.7	-	4.6	29	120	90	0.2	-	-	-	0.1
Channa cow	57.1	18.3	20.8	2.6	-	1.2	265	208	138	-	366	0.07	0.02	-
Channa buffalo	54.1	13.4	23	1.6	-	7.9	292	480	277	-	-	-	-	-
Cheese	40.3	24.1	25.1	4.2	-	6.3	348	790	520	2.1	273	-	-	-
Kheer	69	6.9	12.2	2.3	-	9.6	176	388	237	-	242	0.12	0.35	0.3
Khoa buffalo whole	30.6	14.6	31.2	3.1	-	20.5	421	650	420	5.8	-	-	-	-
Khoa buffalo skim	46.1	22.3	1.6	4.3	-	25.7	206	990	650	2.7	-	-	-	-
Khoa cow	25.2	20	25.9	4	-	24.9	413	956	613	-	497	0.23	0.41	0.4

Continued

Milk and Milk Products

Name of the food	Moisture (gm)	Protein (gm)	Fat (gm)	Minerals (gm)	Fibre (gm)	Carbohydrates (gm)	Energy (kcal)	Calcium (mg)	Phosphorus (mg)	Iron (mg)	Carotene (mg)	Thiamine (mg)	Riboflavin (mg)	Niacin (mg)
Skim milk powder (cowmilk)	4.1	38	0.1	6.8	-	51	357	1370	1000	1.4	0	0.45	1.64	1
Whole milk powder (cowmilk)	3.5	25.8	26.7	6	-	38	496	950	730	0.6	1400	0.31	1.36	0.8

Fats and Oils

Name of the food	Moisture (gm)	Protein (gm)	Fat (gm)	Minerals (gm)	Fibre (gm)	Carbohydrates (gm)	Energy (kcal)	Calcium (mg)	Phosphorus (mg)	Iron (mg)	Carotene (mg)	Thiamine (mg)	Riboflavin (mg)	Niacin (mg)
Butter	19	-	81	2.5	-	-	729	-	-	-	3200	-	-	-
Ghee cow milk	-	-	100	-	-	-	900	-	-	-	2000	-	-	-
Ghee buffalo milk	-	-	100	-	-	-	900	-	-	-	900	-	-	-
Vanaspati	-	-	100	-	-	-	900	-	-	-	2500	-	-	-
Cooking oil	-	-	100	-	-	-	900	-	-	-	0	-	-	-

Source: Nutrient Composition of Indian Foods. NIN, ICMR, 1989.

References

- Gopalan, C., Rama, Sastri, B.V., Balasubramaniam, S.C. 1989, *Nutritive Value of Indian Foods*. Revised and updated by Narasinga, Rao, B.S., Deosthala, Y.G., and Pant, K.C. National Institute of Nutrition, Indian Council of Medical Research, Hyderabad.
- ICMR. 1989. *Nutritive value of Indian Foods*. National Institute of Nutrition, Hyderabad.
- Joshi, S. 2002. *Nutrition and Dietetics*. 2nd edition. Tata McGraw-Hill Publishing Company Limited.
- Khanna, K. 2003. *Textbook of Nutrition and Dietetics*, University of Delhi.
- Kathleen, M.L. *Krause's food, Nutrition, and Diet Therapy*, 9th edition.
- Pansky, B., *Dynamic Anatomy and Physiology*, Macmillan Publishing Co. Inc., New York, 1975.
- Rajalakshmi, K., 1981. *Applied Nutrition*. 3rd edition. IBH Publishing Company.
- Robinson, C.H., Lawler, M.N.1986. *Normal and Therapeutic Nutrition*. 17th edition. Macmillan Publishing Company, New York.
- WHO. 1978, *Arterial Hypertention*. Technical report series 628. WHO, Geneva, pp. 58.

Other Books on
EDUCATION

1.	History of Medieval India **(New)**	495/-
2.	Methodology of Educational Research **(New)**	250/-
3.	Philosophical & Sociological Foundations of Education **(New)**	225/-
4.	Research Methods in Education **(New)**	225/-
5.	Psychology of Learning & Human Development **(New)**	225/-
6.	A New Approach to Teacher & Education in the Emerging Indian Society **(New)**	225/-
7.	Safety and Disaster Management **(New)**	225/-
8.	Measurement and Evaluation in Psychology and Education	225/-
9.	Special Education	225/-
10.	Principles of Office Management	195/-
11.	History of Ancient India	395/-
12.	Select World Constitutions	450/-
13.	Environmental Education	195/-
14.	Experimental Psychology	195/-
15.	Teaching of Home Science	195/-
16.	Educational Thought and Practice	195/-
17.	Guidance and Counselling A Manual	195/-
18.	School Organisation and Administration	195/-
19.	Developmental Psychology	195/-
20.	Social Work Theory and Practice	225/-
21.	Modern Education for New Generation	195/-
22.	Advanced Educational Technology	195/-
23.	Comparative Education	195/-
24.	Introduction to Educational Research	175/-
25.	Computer Education	175/-
26.	Teaching of Chemistry	175/-
27.	Teaching of Physics	175/-
28.	Handbook of Journalism & Mass Media	225/-
29.	Advanced Educational Psychology	195/-
30.	Educational Administration & Origanisation Management	195/-
31.	Social Psychology	225/-
32.	Teaching of Commerce	175/-
33.	Educational Development & Technology	195/-
34.	Disaster Management	195/-
35.	Information Technology	195/-
36.	Human Resource Development	195/-
37.	Mass Media Communication Theory & Practice	225/-
38.	Adult Education	195/-
39.	General Psychology	195/-

40.	Distance Education in India	195/-
41.	Teacher Education	195/-
42.	Educational Philosophy	195/-
43.	Science Teaching in Schools	195/-
44.	Indian National Congress	450/-
45.	Indian Polity **(Revised Edition)**	395/-
46.	New Comparative Government **(Revised Edition)**	350/-
	Advanced Study in the History of Modern India	
47.	(Volume-1: 1707-1813)	225/-
48.	(Volume-2: 1813-1920)	325/-
49.	(Volume-3: 1920-1947)	175/-
50.	Handbook of Nutrition & Dietetics	250/-
51.	Development of Education in India	195/-
52.	A Text Book of Environmental Studies	195/-
53.	Teaching of History	175/-
54.	Administrative Thinkers	195/-
55.	Research Methodology	195/-
56.	Curriculum Development	195/-
57.	Teaching of Science	175/-
58.	Teaching of Mathematics	175/-
59.	Principles of Educational &Vocational Guidance	225/-
60.	Child Psychology	195/-
61.	Abnormal Psychology	225/-
62.	Indian Education in Emerging Society	195/-
63.	Human Resource Management	175/-
64.	Higher Education and Global Challenges	195/-
65.	Teaching of Geography	175/-
66.	Teaching of Social Studies	175/-
67.	Teaching of English	175/-
68.	Education for All The Indian Saga	225/-
69.	Value Education in Global Perspective	195/-
70.	Teacher Training	175/-
71.	Public Administration	175/-
72.	Public Relations & Integrated Communications	195/-
73.	Educational Psychology	175/-
74.	Introduction to Educational Technology	225/-
75.	Textbook of Food and Nutrition	175/-

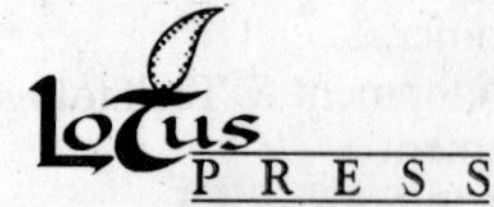

Unit No. 220, 2nd Floor, 4735/22, Prakash Deep Building,
Ansari Road, Darya Ganj, New Delhi- 110002
Ph.: 32903912, 23280047, 9811594448
• E-mail : lotuspress1984@gmail.com, www.lotuspress.co.in